Pancreatic Tumors in Children

Cancer Treatment and Research 8

WILLIAM L. McGUIRE, *series editor*

1. R. B. Livingston, ed., Lung Cancer 1. 1981. ISBN 90-247-2394-9.
2. G. Bennett Humphrey, Louis P. Dehner, Gerald B. Grindey and Ronald T. Acton, eds., Pediatric Oncology 1. 1981. ISBN 90-247-2408-2.
3. Jerome J. DeCosse and Paul Sherlock, eds., Gastrointestinal Cancer 1. 1981. ISBN 90-247-2461-9.
4. John M. Bennett, ed., Lymphomas 1, including Hodgkin's Disease. 1981. ISBN 90-247-2479-1.
5. C. D. Bloomfield, ed., Adult Leukemias 1. 1982. ISBN 90-247-2478-3.
6. D. F. Paulson, ed., Genitourinary Cancer 1. 1982. ISBN 90-247-2480-5.
7. F. M. Muggia, ed., Cancer Chemotherapy 1. 1982. ISBN 90-247-2713-8.

Pancreatic Tumors in Children

edited by

G. BENNETT HUMPHREY
Oklahoma Children's Memorial Hospital and
University of Oklahoma Health Sciences Center

GERALD B. GRINDEY
Lilly Research Laboratories

LOUIS P. DEHNER
University of Minnesota Medical School

RONALD T. ACTON
University of Alabama in Birmingham

THEODORE J. PYSHER
Oklahoma Children's Memorial Hospital and
University of Oklahoma Health Sciences Center

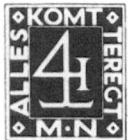

1982

MARTINUS NIJHOFF PUBLISHERS
THE HAGUE / BOSTON / LONDON

Distributors:

for the United States and Canada

Kluwer Boston, Inc.
190 Old Derby Street
Hingham, MA 02043
USA

for all other countries

Kluwer Academic Publishers Group
Distribution Center
P.O. Box 322
3300 AH Dordrecht
The Netherlands

Library of Congress Cataloging in Publication Data CIP

Main entry under title:

Pancreatic tumors in children.

   (Cancer treatment and research ; 8)
   Includes index.
   1. Pancreas--Cancer. 2. Tumors in children.
I. Humphrey, G. Bennett (George Bennett), 1934-
II. Series: Cancer treatment and research ; v. 8.
RC280.P25P37 1983   618.92'99437   82-12626

ISBN-13:978-94-009-7617-7   e-ISBN-13:978-94-009-7615-3
DOI: 10.1007/978-94-009-7615-3

Contents

I. Selected Topics

II. Pancreatic Malignancies

Cancer Treatment and Research

Foreword

Where do you begin to look for a recent, authoritative article on the diagnosis or management of a particular malignancy? The few general oncology textbooks are generally out of date. Single papers in specialized journals are informative but seldom comprehensive; these are more often preliminary reports on a very limited number of patients. Certain general journals frequently publish good in-depth reviews of cancer topics, and published symposium lectures are often the best overviews available. Unfortunately, these reviews and supplements appear sporadically, and the reader can never be sure when a topic of special interest will be covered.

Cancer Treatment and Research is a series of authoritative volumes which aim to meet this need. It is an attempt to establish a critical mass of oncology literature covering virtually all oncology topics, revised frequently to keep the coverage up-to-date, easily available on a single library shelf or by a single personal subscription.

We have approached the problem in the following fashion. First, by dividing the oncology literature into specific subdivisions such as lung cancer, genitourinary cancer, pediatric oncology, etc. Second, by asking eminent authorities in each of these areas to edit a volume on the specific topic on an annual or biannual basis. Each topic and tumor type is covered in a volume appearing frequently and predictably, discussing current diagnosis, staging, markers, all forms of treatment modalities, basic biology, and more.

In Cancer Treatment and Research, we have an outstanding group of editors, each having made a major commitment to bring to this new series the very best literature in his or her field. Martinus Nijhoff Publishers has made an equally major commitment to the rapid publication of high quality books, and world-wide distribution.

Where can you go to find quickly a recent authoritative article on any major oncology problem? We hope that Cancer Treatment and Research provides an answer.

WILLIAM L. MCGUIRE
Series Editor

Preface

'Pancreatic Tumors in Children' is the second volume in the series, 'Cancer Treatment and Research' devoted to pediatric oncology. Like its predecessor, it is organized into two sections. The first section deals with issues of basic research germane to the understanding of human malignancies.

In the second part, major pediatric oncology units in Japan, Australia, Europe and the Americas have been invited to report their experience with an unusual tumor. The topic of this volume is pancreatic carcinoma. The case reports include reviews of the genetics, pathology and diagnostic evaluation of the pediatric pancreatic tumors. However, as there was insufficient experience with chemotherapy and radiotherapy at any one institution, the overview chapter includes recommendations for radiotherapy from Dr. Sarah Donaldson and for chemotherapy from Drs. Philip Schein and Ronald Bukowski. Individuals using these recommended therapies are encouraged to report their results to the editors. That information will then be available to others.

Preface to *Pediatric Oncology 1*

This book is addressed to those who are involved in the care of children with cancer. The editors hope that physicians with training in surgery, radiation therapy, chemotherapy and pathology will find all or some of these articles of interest and pertinence.

The intent of this volume and those to follow is to focus on aspects of pediatric oncology and related fields not consistently and comprehensively covered in other books or journals. Each volume will have two sections. The first section will pursue concepts in research from the basic sciences that the editors feel are applicable to human malignancies. Unique approaches in the clinical management of cancer are also described, as are controversial treatments for specific tumors. We would like to stress that this section will not only report on progress in the treatment of cancer, but will also include topics such as tumor biology, genetics, diagnosis, detection, prevention, psychosocial rehabilitation, etc. All four editors have participated in the planning of this section and all are responsible for its content.

The editors feel that much needs to be learned about specific rare tumors, so it is their intention that the second part of each volume in this series serves as an informal tumor registry with specific malignancies chosen each year. Neoplasms will be selected that occur at a rate such that major centers may encounter only a few examples each year which means that the smaller institution may see one or two cases in a decade. Such low rates of occurrence make treatment difficult since the number of cases does not justify time and effort involved in creating a treatment protocol for each rare tumor; nor do the numbers generate results that will have statistical significance. To compound the problem further, most journals are reluctant to give space to articles reporting fewer than ten patients or in which statistical analysis cannot be undertaken. This inaugural section has taken on the enigmatic problem of the small cell neoplasms in the central nervous system designated by some as the 'primitive neuroectodermal tumor of the CNS.'

In the belief that children and their physicians are bound to benefit from shared knowledge, we have invited some of the major institutions in Japan, Australia, Europe, and the Americas to report their recent experience with specific rare tumors. So that there will be some consistency to the data, we have asked them to limit their reviews to cases treated within the last 10 to 15 years under the assumption that management was probably multimodal and that some of the current antitumor chemotherapeutic agents would have been used. After all the case material was received by the editors, the entire collection was sent back to all participating investigators for their comments. Finally, these have been incorporated by the editors into an overview on the management of that particular tumor group. The editors realize that there are many pitfalls to this approach, primarily caused by inconsistencies in diagnosis and treatment. In spite of these inconsistencies, the editors hope some insight will be gained into the clinical characteristics, overall prognosis, period of greatest risks of relapse for patients who respond to initial therapy, and perhaps also into therapeutic approaches.

In future volumes, a multi-institutional pathological review may be initiated. Two of the editors (GBH, LPD) assume responsibility for this section.

We would like to express our thanks to Dr. William L. McGuire, the series editor, for advice and consultation throughout the preparation of this volume. We would also like to thank Dr. M.L.N. Willoughby, Dr. P.A. Voute, and Dr. Donald Metcalf for serving as consultants to the editors. We would also like to express our thanks to Jeffrey K. Smith, Publisher in the Medical Division of Martinus Nijhoff Publishers for his advice and guidance, and finally to Ms. Lucia Lane and Ms. Leslie Alexander for editorial assistance, and Ms. Terry Kazimir and Ms. Peggy Devinish for secretarial and administrative assistance in preparation of this volume.

We anticipate that *Pediatric Oncology* will be an annual publication. We would like to encourage additional institutions to participate in the recording of rare tumors in the future. Interested parties are encouraged to contact either Dr. Humphrey or Dr. Dehner. All of the editors would also welcome any suggestions for topics that should be reviewed in the future.

List of Editors

HUMPHREY, G. BENNETT, M.D., Ph.D., University of Oklahoma Health Sciences Center, Department of Pediatrics, Hematology-Oncology, Oklahoma Children's Memorial Hospital, P.O. Box 26307, Oklahoma City, OK 73126, U.S.A.

GRINDEY, Dr. Gerald, Lilly Research Laboratories, Department M-305, 307 E. McCarty Street, Indianapolis, IN 46285, U.S.A.

DEHNER, Dr. Louis P., Department of Laboratory Medicine and Pathology, Box 609, Mayo Memorial Building, University of Minnesota Medical School, Minneapolis, MN 55455, U.S.A.

ACTON, Ronald T., Ph.D., Departments of Microbiology & Public Health, University of Alabama in Birmingham, University Station, Birmingham, AL 35294, U.S.A.

PYSHER, Dr. Theodore J., University of Oklahoma Health Sciences Center, Department of Pathology, Oklahoma Children's Memorial Hospital, P.O. Box 26307, Oklahoma City, OK 73126, U.S.A.

List of Contributors

BALABAN, Dr. Gloria B., Department of Pathology/G3, School of Medicine, University of Pennsylvania, 3400 Spruce Street, Philadelphia, PA 19104, U.S.A.

BAUM, Edward S., M.D., Division of Hematology/Oncology, Northwestern University Medical School, Children's Memorial Hospital, 2300 Children's Plaza, Chicago, IL 60614, U.S.A.

BROUGH, A. Joseph, M.D., Department of Laboratory Medicine, Children's Hospital of Michigan, 3901 Beaubien Boulevard, Detroit, MI 48201, U.S.A.

BUKOWSKI, Ronald, M.D., Department of Hematology & Medical Oncology, Cleveland Clinic Foundation, 9500 Euclid Avenue, Cleveland, OH 44106, U.S.A.

CALABRESI, Paul, M.D., Department of Medicine, Roger Williams General Hospital, 825 Chalkstone Avenue, Providence, RI 02908, U.S.A.

CANGIR, Ayten, M.D., Department of Pediatrics, M.D. Anderson Hospital and Tumor Institute, 6723 Bertner Avenue, Houston, TX 77030, U.S.A.

COHN, Isidore, Jr., M.D., Department of Surgery, LSU Medical Center, 1542 Tulane Avenue, New Orleans, LA 70112, U.S.A.

COMPAGNO, John, M.D., CDR, MC, USN, Armed Forces Institute of Pathology, Washington, DC 20306, U.S.A.

CUSHING, Barbara, M.D., Department of Pediatrics, Children's Hospital of Michigan, 3901 Beaubien Boulevard, Detroit, MI 48201, U.S.A.

DEXTER, Dr. Daniel L., Brown University and Roger Williams General Hospital, Department of Medicine, 825 Chalkstone Avenue, Providence, RI 02908, U.S.A.

DONALDSON, Sarah S., M.D., Department of Radiology, Stanford University Medical Center, 300 Pasteur Drive, Stanford, CA 94305, U.S.A.

FALTERMAN, Kenneth W., M.D., Department of Surgery, LSU Medical Center, 1542 Tulane Avenue, New Orleans, LA 70112, U.S.A.

HERBERMAN, Ronald B., M.D., Chief, Laboratory of Immunodiagnosis, National Cancer Institute, NIH, Building 10, Room 8B-02, Bethesda, MD 20205, U.S.A.

HORIE, Akio, M.D., Department of Pathology and Oncology, School of Medicine, University of Occupational and Environmental Health, Yahatanishi-ku, Kitakyushu 807, Japan

HUMPHREY, G. Bennett, M.D., Ph.D., University of Oklahoma Health Sciences Center, Department of Pediatrics, Hematology-Oncology, Oklahoma Children's Memorial Hospital, P.O. Box 26307, Oklahoma City, OK 73126, U.S.A.

JAFFE, Norman, M.D., Department of Pediatrics, M.D. Anderson Hospital and Tumor Institute, 6723 Bertner Avenue, Houston, TX 77030, U.S.A.

KANEKO, Yasuhiko, M.D., Department of Medicine, Box 420, University of Chicago, 950 East 59th Street, Chicago, IL 60637, U.S.A.

KISSANE, John, M.D., Department of Pathology, Washington University Medical School, 660 S. Euclid Avenue, St. Louis, MO 63110, U.S.A.

KROUS, Henry F., M.D., Department of Pathology, Oklahoma Children's Memorial Hospital, P.O. Box 26307, Oklahoma City, OK 73126, U.S.A.

LAMBIRD, Perry, M.D., Pathologist, Medical Arts Laboratory, Pasteur Medical Building, Oklahoma City, OK 73106, U.S.A.

MENDELSOHN, Geoffrey, M.D., Department of Pathology, Johns Hopkins University School of Medicine, Baltimore, MD 21205, U.S.A.

MORGAN, Elaine R., M.D., Division of Hematology/Oncology, Northwestern University Medical School, Children's Memorial Hospital, 2300 Children's Plaza, Chicago, IL 60614, U.S.A.

NOWELL, Peter, M.D., Department of Pathology/G3, School of Medicine, University of Pennsylvania, 3400 Spruce Street, Philadelphia, PA 19104, U.S.A.

OERTEL, James E., M.D., Department of Endocrine Pathology, Armed Forces Institute of Pathology, Washington, DC 20306, U.S.A.

PORTER, Marilyn Gregory, M.D., Department of Pediatrics, Gastroenterology Section, Oklahoma Children's Memorial Hospital, P.O. Box 26307, Oklahoma City, OK 73126, U.S.A.

PYSHER, Theodore J., M.D., Department of Pathology, Oklahoma Children's Memorial Hospital, University of Oklahoma Health Sciences Center, P.O. Box 26307, Oklahoma City, OK 73126, U.S.A.

ROWLEY, Janet D., M.D., Department of Medicine, Box 420, University of Chicago, 950 East 59th Street, Chicago, IL 60637, U.S.A.

SCHEIN, Philip S., M.D., Vincent T. Lombardi Cancer Research Center, Georgetown University Medical Center, 3800 Reservoir Road, N.W., Washington, DC 20007, U.S.A.

SCHIMKE, R. Neil, M.D., F.A.C.P., Professor of Medicine and Pediatrics, Director, Division of Metabolism, Endocrinology and Genetics, Kansas University College of Health Sciences and Hospital, Kansas City, KS 66103, U.S.A.

SCHMIDT, James H., M.D., Associate Director, Adolescent Medicine, Oklahoma Children's Memorial Hospital, University of Oklahoma Health Sciences Center, P.O. Box 26307, Oklahoma City, OK 73126, U.S.A.

SINKS, Lucius F., M.D., Chief, Division of Pediatric and Adolescent Oncology/Hematology, Box 184, New England Medical Center, 171 Harrison Avenue, Boston, MA 02111, U.S.A.

SMITH, E. Ide, M.D., Pediatric Surgery Service, Oklahoma Children's Memorial Hospital, University of Oklahoma Health Sciences Center, P.O. Box 26307, Oklahoma City, OK 73126, U.S.A.

TSUCHIDA, Masahiro, M.D., Department of Pediatrics, Toho University School of Medicine, 6-11-1, Omori-nishi, Otaku, Tokyo, Japan

TSUKIMOTO, Ichiro, M.D., Department of Pediatrics, Toho University School of Medicine, 6-11-1, Omori-nishi, Otaku, Tokyo, Japan

WEEDN, Robert J., M.D., Weedn & Jones Surgical Associates, 111 North 10th Street, Duncan, OK 73533, U.S.A.

WEST, Patrice M., B.S., Division of Hematology/Oncology, Northwestern University Medical School, Children's Memorial Hospital, 2300 Children's Plaza, Chicago, IL 60614, U.S.A.

WILSON, Stuart D., M.D., Division of Surgery, Medical College of Wisconsin, 8700 West Wisconsin Avenue, Milwaukee, WI 53226, U.S.A.

WOO, Shiao Y., MB, MRCP, Division of Pediatric and Adolescent Oncology/Hematology, Box 14, New England Medical Center, 171 Harrison Avenue, Boston, MA 02111, U.S.A.

I. Selected Topics

1. Role of Natural Killer (NK) Cells in Resistance to Tumors

RONALD B. HERBERMAN

Studies on natural cell-mediated cytotoxicity began as a rather restricted effort, to understand a puzzling series of observations that were made during investigations of cell-mediated cytotoxicity in tumor-bearing or in individuals immunized against tumors. The expected finding was specific cytotoxic activity against autologous tumor cells or against tumors of the same histologic or etiologic type. It was assumed in the initial studies that lymphoid cells from normal individuals would be unreactive and thus would serve as good baseline controls for comparison. Indeed, mice or rats immunized against various tumors, especially those induced by type C oncornaviruses, were found to have increased cytotoxic reactivity against the immunizing tumor or against tumor cells sharing the relevant tumor-associated antigens [1–4]. Similarly, a considerable proportion of patients with various types of cancer appeared to selectively react against cell lines derived from tumors of the same organ or of the same histologic type [4, 5].

Although this concept of almost ubiquitous, specific tumor-associated cell-mediated cytotoxicity against tumors became generally accepted, some exceptions to the expected specificity in clinical testing began to be noted by a few investigators. Normal individuals, including those unrelated or unexposed to cancer patients, were found to react against leukemic cells [6] or against cell lines derived from tumors [7–9]. During this period, most investigators in the field attributed this anomalous control reactivity to a variety of *in vitro* artifacts (e.g., see discussion in [10]). However, it was not possible to eliminate the cytotoxic reactivity of normal individuals by technical modifications in the assays. Gradually more and more investigators, including some of those initially describing good cancer patient restricted specificity, reported on cytotoxic reactivity by normal individuals and a lack of complete histologic type-specific reactivity by cancer patients [11–16].

Concurrent with the initial recognition of cytotoxic reactivity by normal human donors were similar observations in rodent systems. When spleen

G. B. Humphrey et al. (eds.), Pancreatic Tumors in Children.
© 1982 Martinus Nijhoff Publishers, The Hague/Boston/London. ISBN-13:978-94-009-7617-7

cells from young, 6–8-week old normal rats were tested as controls for studies of immunity to a Gross virus-induced leukemia, they were found to frequently give substantial levels of lysis above the medium control and often as high as those from tumor-immune rats [17]. Shortly thereafter, similar observations were made with normal mice [18].

Shortly after the phenomenon of natural cell-mediated cytotoxicity was recognized in studies with human and rodent tumor cells, intensive efforts were begun to identify the nature of the responsible lymphoid cells. It was soon found that much of the reactivity was attributable to a particular subpopulation of nonadherent cells, which have been termed NK cells. Within a quite short period of time, studies on NK cells have expanded into a broad and multifaceted research area, ranging from a series of problems in rather fundamental immunobiology to practical issues related to host resistance against tumors and infectious diseases, prognostic indicators, immune surveillance, and immunotherapy. I will here attempt to focus on the possible *in vitro* relevance of NK cells to host resistance against disease. For a more detailed and comprehensive summary of the current state of the field, the reader may refer to a recent book on NK cells and other natural cell-mediated effector mechanisms [19].

1. POSSIBLE IN VIVO ROLES OF NK CELLS

The most important practical issue to be settled is the role of NK cells *in vivo*. Most of the attention has been directed toward the *in vivo* resistance to growth of NK-susceptible tumor cell lines. However, other and potentially more important roles have come up for consideration: a) role in resistance against growth of primary tumors; b) role in immune surveillance against development of spontaneous or carcinogen-induced tumors; c) role in natural resistance against microbial infections; d) role in natural resistance against bone marrow transplants; e) role in graft *versus* host disease; f) role in regulation of differentiation of normal hematopoietic or other cells; and g) role as secretory and immunoregulatory cells. I will here focus on the evidence for a role of NK cells in defenses against tumors.

1.1. Role in Resistance Against Tumor Cell Lines

There is substantial evidence for an important role of NK cells in *in vivo* resistance against established cell lines of tumors, particularly those that show susceptibility to *in vitro* cytolysis by NK cells (summarized in Table 1).

A major approach has been to look for correlations between *in vivo* resistance to the growth of the tumor cell lines and the levels of NK activity in

Table 1. Evidence for *in vivo* role of NK cells against tumor cell lines

---

1. Variations in growth of NK-sensitive cell lines in recipients with different levels of NK activity.
   a. Less growth in nudes than in euthymic mice of same strain.
   b. Less growth in 5–10-week old than in older mice.
   c. Less growth in F_1 hybrids with high NK activity than in those with low activity.
   d. Less growth in radiation chimeras reconstituted with bone marrow from high NK strains.
   e. Increased growth in beige mice.
2. Local and systemic adoptive transfer of resistance to tumor growth, by NK cell-enriched populations.
3. Increased tumor growth in mice treated with anti-asialo GM1.
4. Correlation between *in vivo* elimination of ^{125}IUdR labeled NK-susceptible tumor cells and levels of NK activity in recipients.
   a. More rapid clearance of radioisotope in high NK strains.
   b. More rapid clearance in 4–8-week old mice than in older mice.
   c. Augmentation of clearance in mice with NK activity boosted by interferon, poly I:C, *C. parvum,* pyran or tumor cells.
   d. Depression of clearance in mice with NK activity inhibited by cyclophosphamide, lethal irradiation, corticosteroids, silica, carrageenan, pyran.
   e. Ability to reconstitute both NK activity and *in vivo* clearance in cyclophosphamide-treated mice by intravenous transfer of cells with characteristics of NK cells.

---

the recipients. In several different situations, a good correlation was observed. Some NK-sensitive tumor lines have produced a lower incidence of tumors, and have grown more slowly, in nude or thymectomized mice than in euthymic mice with the same genetic background [20–22]. Fewer transplantable tumors have also been induced in 5–10-week old mice, at the peak of NK activity, than in older mice with low NK activity [20, 23]. Some recent studies have examined the effects of age on growth of several transplantable tumors in nude mice. A much higher incidence of metastases, after either intravenous or subcutaneous transplantation, was seen in 3-week old nude mice, which had low NK activity, than in 6-week old nude mice, which had high NK activity. A high rate of pulmonary metastases in young nude recipients was seen with xenogeneic as well as allogeneic tumor cell lines [24, 25]. Augmentation of NK activity in the 3-week old nude mice, by treatment with poly I:C or *C. parvum,* inhibited the development of metastases. The apparent major role for NK cells in resistance in nude mice against growth of transplantable tumors, and the ability to circumvent this by using nude mice with low NK activity, has practical implications for the strong interest in utilizing nude mice for growth of human tumors. Many investigators have noted the difficulty to grow some tumors in nude mice and the rarity of metastases, even when metastatic deposits of human tumors were transplanted [26-31]. The findings that some human tumor cells are susceptible to mouse NK activity [32, 33] are consistent with a role for NK cells in this resistance.

Kiessling and his associates [34, 35] performed an extensive series of experiments which demonstrated a correlation between the levels of NK activity in different strains of mice and the resistance of F_1 hybrids between each strain and A mice to the A strain lymphoma, YAC, the cultured line of which is highly sensitive to NK activity. Mice which were thymectomized, irradiated, and reconstituted with fetal liver also showed this resistance [21]. Haller et al. [36] extended this approach by transferring bone marrow cells from high or low NK strains to lethally irradiated low NK recipients. Recipients of cells from high NK donors developed high NK activity and had increased resistance to growth of YAC.

The various types of correlations described above have only been observed with tumor lines with some susceptibility to lysis by NK cells. The growth of completely NK-resistant cell lines has not been affected by the levels of NK activity in the recipients (e.g., [22]). It is of interest in this regard that in a study of two sublines of a mouse lung tumor, the metastatic subline was resistant to NK activity, whereas the nonmetastatic subline showed some susceptibility [37].

Beige mice, with low NK activity associated with their recessive point mutation [38], have also provided a convenient model for examining the role of NK cells in resistance to growth of transplantable tumor lines. Talmadge et al. [39] found that an NK-susceptible syngeneic melanoma cell line grew more rapidly and produced more metastases in beige compared to normal mice. This difference was not seen with an NK-resistant subline of the same tumor. Using a similar approach, Karre et al. [40] found that two NK-susceptible syngeneic lymphomas produced a higher incidence of tumors and grew more rapidly in beige than in normal heterozygous littermates.

Another approach to the *in vivo* role of NK cells in the growth of transplantable tumors has been the attempt to transfer increased resistance by NK cell-enriched populations. Kasai et al. [41] enriched for Ly 5+ spleen cells and depleted Thy 1+ and B cells and showed that this small subpopulation of cells had high NK activity. Mixture of these Ly 5+ cells with an NK-sensitive lymphoma cell line resulted in reduced tumor incidence after transplantation. Similarly, local adoptive transfer of cells bearing the NK-1 antigen, and thereby enriched for NK activity, suppressed growth of the YAC lymphoma [42]. Systemic adoptive transfer of cells, with the characteristics of NK cells, from normal or nude mice, was also found, in an immunochemotherapy model system, to increase protection against a transplantable leukemia [43].

In an alternative approach that utilized information about selective markers on mouse NK cells, Habu *et al.* [44] administered anti-asialo GM1 to nude mice. The treated mice had almost no detectable NK activity and showed increased susceptibility to transplantation of syngeneic, allogeneic and human tumors.

Although the above studies point to a significant role of NK cells in resistance against tumor growth, they do not conclusively show that NK cells are the actual *in vivo* effector cells. Since these studies relied on measurement of tumor incidence or growth rate, at a considerable time after tumor challenge, one cannot rule out the possibility that NK cells helped to induce or recruit other effector mechanisms, such as T cells or activated macrophages. To obtain more direct information about the role of NK cells in the direct and rapid *in vivo* elimination of tumor cells, ^{125}I-iododeoxyuridine (^{125}IUdR) labeled tumor cells were inoculated intravenously and clearance from the lungs and other organs was measured [45–47]. In young mice of strains with high NK activity, there was a greater clearance of radioactivity when measured at 2–4 hours after inoculation than was seen in strains with low reactivity. In parallel with the decline of NK activity in mice after 10–12 weeks of age, *in vivo* clearance of intravenously inoculated tumor cells was also found to decrease. Furthermore, treatment of mice with a variety of agents that produced augmented or decreased *in vitro* reactivity also resulted in similar shifts in *in vivo* reactivity (Table 1). Such correlations were observed with several NK-susceptible tumor lines and not with some completely NK-resistant lines [46].

As further confirmation of the role of NK cells in resistance to growth of NK-susceptible transplantable tumors, transfer of NK cell-containing populations into mice with cyclophosphamide-induced depression of NK activity was shown to significantly restore both *in vivo* clearance and NK reactivity [48, 49]. The effectiveness of the transfer correlated with the levels of NK activity of donor cells in a variety of situations: a) NK-reactive spleen cells were able to transfer reactivity whereas NK-unreactive thymus cells were ineffective; b) spleen cells from young mice of high NK strains were considerably more effective than cells from older mice or from strains with low NK activity; c) the cells responsible for transfer had the characteristics of NK cells, being nonadherent, nonphagocytic, expressing asialo GM1 and lacking easily detectable Thy 1 antigen; and d) cells from donors with drug-induced depression of NK activity were unable to transfer reactivity. These results extend the recent findings of Hanna and Fidler [50], who showed that the transfer of NK-reactive spleen cells to cyclophosphamide-treated mice could decrease the number of metastases developing in the lungs after challenge with NK-susceptible solid tumor cells.

A similar pattern of results was obtained when radiolabeled cells were inoculated subcutaneously into the footpads of mice [51]. Clearance correlated in several ways with the levels of NK activity in the recipients and cells with the characteristics of NK cells were effective in local adoptive transfer. However, in contrast to NK activity and the results with intravenously inoculated tumor cells, no decrease in clearance was observed in older or beige mice. Those results suggest that other effector cells may also be involved in reactivity in subcutaneous tissues (e.g., the natural cytotoxic cells described by Stutman *et al.* [52, 53]) or that in some situations local factors may augment the NK cell activity.

Although the results in some studies, particularly those with intravenously inoculated radiolabeled tumor cells, suggested that NK cells may be particularly involved in resistance against hematogenous metastatic spread of tumors [50], the results with the footpad assay [51] and the various demonstrations of NK-related differences in outgrowth of subcutaneous tumors indicate that natural effector cells can also enter and be active at sites of local tumor growth. This is supported by the direct demonstration of NK cells in cell suspensions prepared from small tumors growing at subcutaneous or intramuscular locations [54]. Thus, NK cells have the potential to be involved in the primary line of defense against both the local outgrowth as well as the metastatic spread of transplanted tumors. However, it appears that the effectiveness of this natural resistance mechanism is rather limited. Even with tumor cells that are highly susceptible to NK activity, development of progressively growing tumors can occur in animals with high NK activity. The mechanisms for such escape from complete elimination by NK cells are not clear, but the possible explanations include: a) development of resistance of the tumor cells to lysis by NK cells. NK-susceptible cultured tumor lines have been shown to become relatively NK-resistant after growth *in vivo* [55, 56]. The nature of this resistance is not well defined, but there have been some indications that it is reversible [55]. Treatment of some NK-resistant cell lines with inhibitors of RNA or protein synthesis has been found to make them sensitive to lysis by NK cells [57, 58]. Interferon has been found to be one of the mediators of induction of NK-resistance of target cells, since pretreatment of some NK-sensitive target cells with interferon can render them resistant [59, 60]; b) inhibition of NK activity in tumor-bearing individuals. Tumor-bearing mice [61, 62] and cancer patients with advanced disease [63–67] have been found to have low NK activity. This may be due, at least in part, to the development of suppressor cells. Cell suspensions prepared from large tumors in mice [68] and from some human tumors [54, 69–71] have been shown to contain macrophages or other lymphoid cells which could inhibit NK activity. Prostaglandin production by such suppressor cells or by the tumor cells might be responsible for some of the depressed NK activity, since treatment of mice bearing murine sarcoma virus-induced tumors with inhibitors of prostaglandin synthesis (indomethacin or aspirin) partially or completely restored NK activity to normal levels [72].

1.2. Role in Resistance Against Growth of Primary Tumors

From the available evidence that was summarized above, it seems likely that NK cells play an important role in resistance to growth and metastatic spread of some tumor cell lines. Although such results are encouraging, they do not indicate whether NK cells also can have a similar role in defense against growth and metastasis of primary tumors. To obtain evidence in support of such a fraction, it would be desirable to document the following predictions: a) primary tumor cells should have some demonstrable susceptibility to recognition by NK cells; b) the NK cells of tumor-bearing individuals should be able, under some circumstances, to interact with the autologous tumor; c) selective alterations in NK activity in tumor-bearing individuals should affect the growth or degree of metastatic spread of the tumors.

Unfortunately, information relevant to any of these points is quite scanty and, to my knowledge, no clear data exist for the last prediction. Before reviewing the available evidence regarding NK reactivity against primary tumor cells, I would like to point out the difficulties that would be anticipated were NK cells playing a significant role in growth of primary tumors. For such studies, one would have to obtain tumors of sufficient size to prepare adequate numbers of tumor cells. By definition, such tumors had to have been at least relatively successful in evading host defense mechanisms. Therefore, if NK cells play an important role in resistance, one would predict that tumor outgrowth would only occur in the face of relative resistance to lysis by NK cells and/or depression of NK activity. Thus, the data most consistent with these qualifications of the earlier stated predictions would be detectable but low levels of interaction between NK cells and tumor cells.

As summarized in Table 2, some evidence has been accumulated in this

Table 2. Evidence for reactivity of NK cells against primary tumors

1. Low levels of susceptibility of some primary tumors to lysis by NK cells.
   Mouse: AKR lymphomas, C3H mammary tumors
   Human: Some leukemias, carcinomas, and other tumors
2. Cold target inhibition of NK activity by some primary mouse and human tumors.
3. *In situ* localization of mouse NK cells in small spontaneous mammary tumors and in primary murine sarcoma virus-induced tumors.
4. Low levels of NK reactivity of syngeneic, and even autologous tumor-bearing individuals, against some primary tumor cells.

direction. The majority of spontaneous mammary tumors of C3H mice [73] and of spontaneous lymphomas in AKR mice [74] have been found to have detectable, albeit low, susceptibility to lysis by NK cells. Similarly, some human leukemias [6, 75, 76], a myeloma [75], and some carcinomas, sarcomas, and melanomas [77, 78] have been significantly lysed by NK cells. Such lysis has been appreciably augmented, and thereby evident with a higher proportion of tumors, when the effector cells were pretreated with interferon [75–78]. As further support for the ability of NK cells to recognize primary tumor cells, Ortaldo *et al.* [79] showed that a variety of human tumor cells could cold target inhibit the lysis of radiolabeled K562 cells. Most of these positive results were obtained with NK cells from normal allogeneic donors. In fact, Vánky *et al.* [77] detected NK reactivity only against allogeneic human tumor cells and concluded that the NK cells of the tumor-bearing individual lacked the ability to recognize the autologous tumor cells. They postulated that recognition of foreign histocompatibility antigens was involved in lysis by NK cells, particularly those stimulated by interferon. If correct, their hypothesis would virtually preclude a role for NK cells in resistance against primary tumor growth. However, such restriction of NK reactivity to allogeneic tumors does not fit the many examples of tumor cell lines being susceptible to syngeneic NK cells (e.g., [61, 80]). Similarly, normal C3H mice have been found to be reactive against some syngeneic mammary tumors [73], and some cancer patients also have had detectable, interferon-augmentable, NK activity against their autologous tumor cells [78]. The reasons for the discrepancies among the human studies are not clear. The positive results were obtained with ovarian carcinoma cells, mainly in 20-hr cytotoxicity assays [78], whereas the allo-restricted results involved other types of tumors, tested only in 4-hr assays. The greater sensitivity of the prolonged assay would seem sufficient to account for the differences. In addition, it is possible that the subpopulation of NK cells that are required to interact to certain types of tumors may be selectively inhibited in the autologous tumor-bearing host.

Another line of evidence in support of the possibility for NK cells to interact *in vivo* with autologous primary tumor cells is the demonstration that NK cells can enter and accumulate at the site of tumor growth. NK cells have been detected in small spontaneous mouse mammary carcinomas [54] and in small primary mouse tumors induced by murine sarcoma virus [54, 81]. In contrast, NK activity has usually been undetectable in large tumors in mice [54] or in clinical tumor specimens. This may be due, at least in part, to the presence of suppressor cells, which have been demonstrated in some cell suspensions from some tumors [54, 68–71].

To further support the possible role of NK cells in resistance against the growth of primary tumors, it would be very helpful to examine the effects of selective alterations of NK activity in tumor-bearers. However, very few experiments specifically designed to examine this issue have been reported. Suggestive evidence has come from the administration of indomethacin to mice bearing primary murine sarcoma virus-induced tumors [72]. With a treatment schedule that augmented the depressed NK reactivity, tumor incidence and size were reduced and a higher proportion of tumors completely regressed. Similarly, one could invoke the therapeutic efficacy of interferon for some primary tumors, a treatment known to augment NK reactivity. The limitations of such data are that such agents have pleiotropic effects and it is not possible to determine whether the alterations in other functions had the more important influence on tumor growth. Studies with more selective alterations in NK activity will be needed to settle this issue. Such experiments probably should be performed in individuals with only a small amount of tumor present, to allow the detection of effects on tumor growth that might be more likely during a phase when the host is not already overwhelmed by extensive tumor burden.

1.3. Role in Immune Surveillance Against Tumors

Of paramount interest is whether NK cells may be involved in immune surveillance against the initial development of spontaneous or carcinogen-induced tumors. Such a consideration is particularly pertinent at this time, since the whole concept of immune surveillance is being questioned [82, 83]. The original formulations of the immune surveillance hypothesis emphasized the central importance of the immune system in prevention of spontaneous tumors [84, 85]. Later, the theory was modified to stress the key role of thymus-dependent immunity in immune surveillance [86]. The frequent, recent criticisms of the hypothesis have focused on two main issues: a) the inability of the modified theory to account for a number of observations in T cell-deficient mice. For example, much attention has been given to the decreased incidence of mouse mammary tumors in neonatally thymectomized mice and to the failure to observe more rapid tumor growth or even higher incidences of spontaneous or chemical carcinogen-induced tumors in nude mice [87, 88]; b) the failure to find evidence for tumor-associated transplantation antigens on many spontaneous tumors [89]. The latter problem has led to the suggestion that immune surveillance may only be operative against tumors induced by oncogeneic viruses, which usually have strong transplantation antigens [90]. The major exceptions to the central role of immune T cells in resistance to tumor development has led many investigators to more generally question the theory of immune surveillance. Even a counter-theory of immuno-stimulation has been formulated [91], suggesting that the immune system may have mainly enhancing effects on tumor induction and growth.

Postulation of an important role of NK cells in immune surveillance offers possible solutions for both of the major difficulties with the theory. The observations that nude or neonatally thymectomized mice or rats have high levels of NK activity would then be compatible with their relatively low incidence of tumors. Furthermore, susceptibility of tumor cells to attack by NK cells seems to be independent of the expression of tumor-associated transplantation antigens, thus leaving open the possibility for surveillance against tumors lacking such classically defined and immune T cell-dependent antigens.

Given such attractive theoretical arguments for the possible participation of NK cells in immune surveillance, what then is the available supportive evidence? Thus far, very few well-designed experiments have been performed to directly address this issue. However, before turning to those, it is of interest to summarize several pieces of circumstantial evidence that are consistent with, or suggestive of, a role for NK cells (Table 3). 1) NK activity has been shown to be substantially augmented by retinoic acid [92], which has been reported to retard the development of some primary tumors [93]. In support of this possibility, cells with the characteristics of NK cells have been found to inhibit the *in vitro* proliferation of autologous EBV-infected B cells [94]. 2) Patients with the genetically determined Chediak-Higashi syndrome have a high risk of development of lymphoproliferative diseases [95]. In recent detailed studies on several patients with this disease [96, 97], all were found to have profound deficits in NK and K cell activities, whereas a variety of other immune functions, including cytotoxicity against tumor cells by T cells, monocytes and granulocytes, was essentially normal. 3) Similarly, beige mice, which have an analogous genetic defect, also have a substantial [38, 98], but incomplete [99, 100], selective

Table 3. Circumstantial evidence for a role of NK cells in immune surveillance

1. High NK activity in nude or neonatally thymectomized consistent with their low incidence of spontaneous mammary tumors or chemical carcinogen-induced tumors.
2. Augmentation of NK activity by retinoic acid, a tumor preventive agent, and inhibition of NK activity by tumor promoters.
3. High incidence of lymphoproliferative diseases in patients with Chediak-Higashi syndrome, who have a selective deficit in NK activity.
4. High incidence of lymphomas in a colony of beige mice, which also have a selective deficit in NK activity.
5. Low NK activity in patients with X-linked lymphoproliferative disease.
6. Low NK activity in kidney allograft recipients, who have a high risk of development of lymphoproliferative and other tumors.

deficiency in NK activity. A small colony of aged beige mice have recently been reported to have a high incidence of lymphomas [101]. 4) Another human genetic abnormality, X-linked lymphoproliferative disease [102], has been associated with a defect in the ability to control proliferation of B cells infected with Epstein-Barr virus (EBV). Recently, low NK activity has been found in such individuals and this deficit has been suggested to be involved in the pathogenesis of the disease [103]. 5) Patients on immunosuppressive therapy after kidney allotransplants have a high risk of developing tumors, both reticuloendothelial tumors and also a variety of carcinomas [104]. Patients on such treatment regimens have recently been found to have very low NK activity and this has been suggested as a contributing factor to the subsequent development of tumors [105]. Each of these lines of evidence fits one of the major predictions of the immune surveillance theory, that tumor development would be associated with, and in fact preceded by, depressed immunity.

A related prediction of the immune surveillance theory is that carcinogenic agents would cause depressed immune function, thereby impairing the ability of the host to reject the transformed cells. This postulate has been examined by many investigators in regard to the possible role of mature T cells and humoral immunity, and conflicting results have been obtained [87]. In contrast, the initial and still fragmentary data on this point in relation to NK cells are promising. 1) Urethane, which produces lung tumors in only some strains of mice, caused transient and marked depression of NK activity in a susceptible strain [106] but not in resistant strains [107]. Administration of normal bone marrow cells, which as discussed earlier can reconstitute NK activity, to urethane-treated mice reduced the subsequent development of lung tumors ([108]; Gorelik and Herberman, unpublished observations). Also, infection during the latent period with various viruses, each known to induce interferon and thereby augment NK activity, also reduced the incidence of lung tumors induced by urethane. 2) Carcinogenic doses of dimethylbenzanthracene also were found to produce depression of NK activity during the latent period [109]. 3) Sublethal irradiation of mice has been found to cause considerable depression of NK activity [110]. Of particular interest, the schedule of multiple, low doses of irradiation of C57BL mice, that has been highly effective in inducing leukemia in this strain, was found to produce a substantial deficit in NK activity ([111]; Gorelik and Herberman, unpublished observations). The depressed NK activity could be restored by transfer of normal bone marrow cells (Gorelik and Herberman, unpublished observations), a procedure which has been reported to interfere with radiation-induced leukogenesis [112]. 4) NK activity also has been strongly inhibited by two different classes of potent tumor promoters, phorbol esters [92, 113] and teleocidin

(Goldfarb, Sugimura, and Herberman, unpublished observations). All of these observations support the possibility that one of the requisites for tumor induction by carcinogenic agents may be interference with host defenses, including those mediated by NK cells.

Further studies are needed to more directly demonstrate a role for NK cells in immune surveillance. Ideally, one would like to show increased tumorigenesis when NK activity is selectively depressed and reduced tumor formation when such deficiencies are selectively reconstituted or normal levels of reactivity are selectively augmented. However, there are several practical problems which limit vigorous pursuit of such experimental protocols. In addition to the long periods of time needed for such studies and difficulties in identifying the most relevant experimental carcinogenesis models, completely selective and sustained alterations of NK activity are not easily found or-produced. For example, as discussed above, much attention is currently being given to the beige mouse model, as a test system for oncogenesis in NK-deficient animals. However, beige mice have some residual NK activity, which can be augmented by interferon [99] and which can approach normal levels upon prolonged incubations with target cells [100]. Furthermore, they appear to have normal levels of natural cytotoxic activity *in vitro* against some monolayer tumor target cells [114] and *in vivo* against subcutaneous inoculations of both lymphoma and carcinoma cell lines [51]. In addition, the rate of cytotoxicity by macrophages is also somewhat retarded [115], so that an increased tumor incidence in beige mice could not be definitively attributed to the deficit in NK activity. Conversely, induction of interferon or other procedures to augment NK activity generally also alter other immune functions. Yet another, and perhaps the most central, limitation to the use of beige mice or other NK deficient mice to evaluate the role of NK cells in prevention of carcinogenesis is that, as discussed above, many of the carcinogens themselves can strongly inhibit NK activity. Thus, after treatment with a carcinogen, the normal recipients may have as low NK activity as the beige mice and therefore differences in tumor development might not be seen. The most convincing protocol might be to reconstitute animals with depressed NK activity, by adoptive transfer of purified NK cells, and determine the effects on carcinogenesis.

2. CLINICAL CORRELATIONS

One major issue of practical importance has been whether measurement of NK activity in cancer patients would provide information that could help in the management of the disease. Depressed NK activity has been observed in mice [61, 62] and patients [63–67] bearing various types of tumors, and this has been particularly associated with large tumor burdens. This raises the possibility that determination of NK activity in cancer patients might have prognostic value and studies to directly address this question seem warranted. Depressed NK activity has also been associated with other diseases, e.g., active multiple sclerosis [116] and systemic lupus erythematosus [117], and thus this parameter may have more general clinical applicability.

Another aspect of potential clinical importance is the possible effects of therapy on NK activity. This is of interest from two different standpoints. On the one hand, various forms of conventional therapy might inhibit NK activity and thereby have potentially deleterious effects on resistance against tumor growth. On the other hand, some treatments could actually cause an augmentation of NK activity and such an effect might contribute to the therapeutic efficacy of the agent. NK activity in mice and rats has been found to be relatively but not completely resistant to high doses of radiation [118–120]. Even when investigators have found little or no effect on NK activity shortly after radiation, a later and relatively prolonged depression in reactivity was seen [110]. In regard to chemotherapeutic agents, mouse or rat NK cells have been shown to be quite sensitive to cyclophosphamide, hydrocortisone, and some other agents [119, 120]. However, these agents did not interfere with boosting of NK activity by poly I:C, suggesting the existence of treatment-resistant pre-NK cells. On a clinical level, there is a surprising paucity of information on the effects of radiotherapy or chemotherapy on NK activity. The few reports that have dealt with this issue have suggested some but not impressive treatment-related decreases in activity [9, 66, 67, 121]. There is almost no information on the ability of interferon or other agents to boost the depressed reactivity of treated patients, and as a possible analogy to the rodent data, this would seem to be quite worthwhile to examine. In fact, one report has indicated that cyclosporin A strongly inhibited human NK activity but had no effect on boosting by interferon [122]. It should be noted that some chemotherapeutic agents have not depressed NK activity [120, 123] and others, depending on the route and dosage, could induce either increased or decreased reactivity. Adriamycin has been shown to fall into this last category. Initial studies indicated that this drug had little or no inhibitory effect on NK activity [120, 123]. However, a later, more detailed study indicated that adriamycin could depress splenic NK activity, apparently due to the activation of suppressor macrophages, whereas it led to a substantial augmentation of NK activity in the peritoneal cavity, bone marrow, and lymph nodes [124].

3. IMPLICATIONS FOR IMMUNOTHERAPY

Given the possible important role of NK cells in resistance against growth of primary tumors, one possible approach to immunotherapy of cancer is to attempt to restore NK function in tumor-bearers with depressed activity or even to augment reactivity above spontaneous levels. In parallel, one would expect to also augment ADCC activity, since the effector cells appear to be in overlapping subpopulations [125-127] and treatments which stimulate NK activity also increase ADCC [128]. To fully exploit this rationale, it seems important to develop protocols for optimal and sustained augmentation of these cytotoxic functions and then utilize such protocols for clinical immunotherapy. These considerations are particularly pertinent in regard to the current interest in therapy with interferon. Treatment of lymphoid cells [129-132] or purified NK cells [133] with IFN-inducers or IFN, including pure preparations of human IFN [134, 135], has been shown to cause an appreciable augmentation in NK activity. As a result of many studies, it appears that IFN plays a central role in activating or augmenting the activity of NK cells. Most agents which can boost NK activity, either *in vivo* or *in vitro*, appear to be acting by their ability to induce IFN. Conversely, most biological response modifiers in current use or consideration for immunotherapy of cancer have been shown to induce IFN and augment NK activity [136]. The ability of IFN to appreciably augment NK and ADCC activities may provide a rationale for its antitumor effects and may also provide a basis for developing better protocols for therapy with IFN. The current therapeutic protocols with IFN or IFN-inducers are essentially empirical, involving frequent, often daily, administration of very high doses, close to or at the limits of tolerable toxicity. The protocol for optimal and sustained augmentation of NK and ADCC activities may be quite far from the current regimens, and it seems possible that such an alternative protocol could have greater therapeutic efficacy. Determination of an optimal protocol for augmentation of NK activity is of particular concern for some of the IFN-inducers, since they not only have the potential to augment NK activity but also to depress it, via induction or activation of suppressor cells [137].

Another strategy to consider in regard to altering the depressed NK activity of tumor-bearing individuals relates to the possibility that this may be due, at least in part, to the presence of suppressor cells and/or elevated production of prostaglandins. As already mentioned earlier, in at least one animal tumor model, the presence of suppressor cells and elevated production of prostaglandins have been incriminated as factors in the progression of tumor growth. Primary tumors induced in mice by murine sarcoma virus contained suppressor cells when growing progressively but not under conditions when regression occurred [54, 68]. Elevated prostaglandin levels have also been detected in mice bearing these tumors [138, 139]. Treatment of virus-inoculated mice with indomethacin or aspirin, which inhibit prostaglandin synthesis, resulted in restoration of normal levels of NK activity [72] and in suppression of tumor development and growth [72, 138]. Such findings may have more general relevance. Administration of prostaglandins has been found to facilitate carcinogenesis in mice by methylcholanthrene [140] and indomethacin or aspirin have been shown to reduce the growth of several experimental tumors or to augment the antitumor effects of some immunostimulants [139, 141, 142]. The possible mediation of these effects by alterations in the function of NK cells is an attractive hypothesis and may provide a rational basis for the antitumor effects of inhibitors of prostaglandin synthesis. Monitoring levels of NK activity in tumor-bearers receiving such agents may help to determine optimal treatment schedules.

REFERENCES

1. Oren ME, Herberman RB, Canty TG: Immune response to Gross virus-induced lymphoma. II. Kinetics of the cellular immune response. J Natl Cancer Inst 46:621–629, 1971.
2. Leclerc JC, Gomard E, Levy JP: Cell-mediated reaction against tumors induced by oncornaviruses. I. Kinetics and specificity of the immune response in murine sarcoma virus (MSV)-induced tumors and transplanted lymphomas. Int J Cancer 10:589–601, 1972.
3. Lavrin DH, Herberman RB, Nunn M, Soares N: in vitro cytotoxicity studies of murine sarcoma virus (MSV)-induced immunity in mice. J Natl Cancer Inst 51:1497–1508, 1973.
4. Herberman RB: Cell-mediated immunity to tumor cells. In: Advances in cancer research, Vol. 19, Klein G, Weinhouse S (eds). New York: Academic Press, 1974, pp. 207–263.
5. Hellström KE, Hellström J: Lymphocyte-mediated cytotoxicity and blocking serum activity to tumor antigens. Adv Immunol 18:209–277, 1974.
6. Rosenberg EB, Herberman RB, Levine PH, Halterman RH, McCoy JL, Wunderlich JR: Lymphocyte cytotoxicity reactions to leukemia-associated antigens in identical twins. Int J Cancer 9:648–658, 1972.
7. Oldham RK, Herberman RB: Evaluation of cell-mediated cytotoxic reactivity against tumor associated antigens, utilizing ^{125}I-iododeoxyuridine labeled target cells. J Immunol 111:1862–1871, 1973.
8. McCoy JL, Herberman RB, Rosenberg EB, Donnelly FC, Levine PH, Alford C: ^{51}Chromium-release assay for cell-mediated cytotoxicity of human leukemia and lymphoid tissue-culture cells. Natl Cancer Inst Monogr 37:59–67, 1973.
9. Rosenberg EB, McCoy JL, Green SS, Donnelly FC, Siwarski DF, Levine PH, Herberman RB: Destruction of human lymphoid tissue culture cell lines by human peripheral blood lymphocytes in ^{51}Cr-release cellular cytotoxicity assays. J Natl Cancer Inst 52:345, 1974.
10. Herberman RB, Gaylord CE (eds): Conference and workshop on cellular immune reactions to human tumor-associated antigens. Natl Cancer Inst Monogr 37:1–221, 1973.

11. Takasugi M. Mickey MR, Terasaki PI: Reactivity of normal lymphocytes from normal persons on cultured tumor cells. Cancer Res 33:2898–2902, 1973.

12. Skurzak HM, Steiner L, Klein E, Lamon EW: Cytotoxicity of human peripheral lymphocytes for glioma, osteosarcoma and glia cell lines. Natl Cancer Inst Monogr 37:93–99, 1973.

13. Heppner G, Henry E, Stolbach L, Cummings F, McDonough E, Calabresi P: Problems in the clinical use of the microcytotoxicity assay for measuring cell-mediated immunity to tumor cells. Cancer Res 35:1931–1937, 1975.

14. Peter HH, Kalden JR, Seeland P, Diehl V, Eckert G: Humoral and cellular immune reactions in vitro against allogeneic and autologous melanoma cells. Clin Exp Immunol 20:193–207, 1975.

15. Kay HD, Thota H, Sinkovics JG: A comparative study on in vitro cytotoxic reactions of lymphocytes from normal donors and patients with sarcomas to cultured tumor cells. Clin Immunol Immunopathol 5:218–234, 1976.

16. Canevari S, Fossati G, DellaPorta G: Cellular immune reaction to human malignant melanoma and breast carcinoma cells. J Natl Cancer Inst 56:705–709, 1976.

17. Nunn M, Djeu J, Lavrin D, Herberman R: Natural cytotoxic reactivity of rat lymphocytes against syngeneic Gross leukemia. Proc Am Assoc Cancer Res 14:87, 1973.

18. Herberman RB, Ting CC, Kirchner H, Holden H, Glaser M, Bonnard GD, Lavrin D: Effector mechanisms in tumour immunity. In: Progress in immunology, II, Brent L, Holborow J (eds). Amsterdam: North-Holland Publishing Co, 1974, pp. 285–295.

19. Herberman RB (ed): Natural cell-mediated immunity against tumors. New York: Academic Press, 1980.

20. Herberman RB, Holden HT: Natural cell-mediated immunity. Adv Cancer Res 27: 305–377, 1978.

21. Kiessling R, Petrányi G, Klein G, Wigzell H: Non-T-cell resistance against a mouse Moloney lymphoma. Int J Cancer 17:275–281, 1976.

22. Riesenfeld I, Orn A, Gidlund M, Axberg I, Alm GV, Wigzell H: Positive correlation between in vitro NK activity and in vivo resistance towards AKR lymphoma cells. Int J Cancer 25:399–403, 1980.

23. Sendo F, Aoki T, Boyse EA, Buofo CK: Natural occurrence of lymphocytes showing cytotoxic activity to BALB/c radiation-induced leukemia RLOL cells. J Natl Cancer Inst 55:603–609, 1975.

24. Hanna N: Expression of metastatic potential of tumor cells in young nude mice is correlated with low levels of natural killer cell-mediated cytotoxicity. Int J Cancer 26:675–680, 1980.

25. Hanna N, Fidler IJ: Expression of metastatic potential of allogenic and xenogeneic neoplasms in young nude mice. Cancer Res 41:438–444, 1981.

26. Rygaard J, Poulsen CO: Heterotransplantation of a human malignant tumor to nude mice. Acta Pathol Microbiol Scand 77:759–760, 1969.

27. Castro JE: Human tumours grown in mice. Nature New Biol 239:83–84, 1972.

28. Ozzello L, Sordat B, Merenda C, Carrel S, Hurlimann J, Mach JP: Transplantation of a human mammary carcinoma cell line (BT 20) into nude mice. J Natl Cancer Inst 52:1669–1672, 1974.

29. Schmidt M, Good RA: Cancer xenografts in nude mice. Lancet 1:39, 1976.

30. Maguire H Jr, Outzen HC, Custer RP, Prehn RT: Invasion and metastasis of a xenogeneic tumor in nude mice. J Natl Cancer Inst 57:439–442, 1976.

31. Sharkey FE, Fogh J: Metastasis of human tumors in athymic nude mice. Int J Cancer 24:733–738, 1979.

32. Haller O, Kiessling R, Örn A, Kärre K, Nilsson K, Wigzell H: Natural cytotoxicity to

human leukemia mediated by mouse non-T-cells. Int J Cancer 20:93–103, 1977.

33. Nunn ME, Herberman RB: Natural cytotoxicity of mouse, rat and human lymphocytes against heterologous target cells. J Natl Cancer Inst 62:765–771, 1979.

34. Kiessling R, Petrányi G, Klein G, Wigzell H: Genetic variation of *in vitro* cytolytic activity and *in vivo* rejection potential of non-immunized semisyngeneic mice against a mouse lymphoma line. Int J Cancer 15:933–940, 1975.

35. Petrányi G, Kiessling R, Povey S, Klein G, Herzenberg E, Wigzell H: The genetic control of natural killer cell activity and its association with *in vivo* resistance against a Moloney lymphoma isograft. Immunogenetics 3:15–28, 1976.

36. Haller O, Kiessling R, Örn A, Wigzell H: Generation of natural killer cells: an autonomous function of the bone marrow. J Exp Med 145:1411–1416, 1977.

37. Gorelik E, Fogel M, Feldman M, Segal S: Differences in resistance of metastatic tumor cells and cells from local tumor growth to cytotoxicity of natural killer cells. J Natl Cancer Inst 63:1397–1404, 1979.

38. Roder J, Duwe A: The beige mutation in the mouse selectively impairs natural killer cell function. Nature 278:451–453, 1979.

39. Talmadge JE, Meyers KM, Prieur DJ, Starkey JR: Role of NK cells in tumour growth and metastasis in beige mice. Nature 284:622–624, 1980.

40. Kärre K, Klein GO, Kiessling R, Klein G, Roder JC: Low natural *in vivo* resistance to syngeneic leukaemias in natural killer-deficient mice. Nature 284:624–626, 1980.

41. Kasai M, Leclerc JC, McVay-Boudreau L, Shen FW, Cantor H: Direct evidence that natural killer cells in nonimmune spleen cell populations prevent tumor growth *in vivo*. J Exp Med 149:1260–1264, 1979.

42. Tam MR, Emmons SL, Pollack SB: FACS analysis and enrichment of NK effector cells. In: Natural cell-mediated immunity against tumors, Herberman RB (ed). New York: Academic Press, 1980, pp. 265–276.

43. Cheever MA, Greenberg PD, Fefer A: Therapy of leukemia by nonimmune syngeneic spleen cells. J Immunol 124:2137–2142, 1980.

44. Habu S, Fukui H, Shimamura K, Kasai M, Nagai Y, Okumura K, Tamaoki N: *In vivo* effects of anti-asialo GMI. I. Reduction of NK activity and enhancement of transplanted tumor growth in nude mice. J Immunol (in press).

45. Riccardi C, Puccetti P, Santoni A, Herberman RB: Rapid *in vivo* assay of mouse NK cell activity. J Natl Cancer Inst 63:1041-1045, 1979.

46. Riccardi C, Santoni A, Barlozzari T, Puccetti P, Herberman RB: *In vivo* natural reactivity of mice against tumor cells. Int J Cancer 25:475–486, 1980.

47. Riccardi C, Santoni A, Barlozzari T, Herberman RB: Role of NK cells in rapid *in vivo* clearance of radiolabeled tumor cells. In: Natural cell-mediated immunity against tumors, Herberman RB (ed). New York: Academic Press, 1980, pp 1121–1139.

48. Riccardi C, Barlozzari T, Santoni A, Herberman RB, Cesarini C: Transfer to cyclophosphamide-treated mice of natural killer (NK) cells and *in vivo* natural reactivity against tumors. J Immunol 126:1284–1289, 1981.

49. Riccardi C, Santoni A, Barlozzari T, Cesarini C, Herberman RB: *In vivo* role of NK cells against neoplastic or non-neoplastic cells. In: Human cancer immunology. NK cells: Fundamental aspects and role in cancer, Serrou B, Rosenfeld C (eds). Amsterdam: North-Holland Publishing Co, (in press).

50. Hanna N, Fidler IJ: The role of natural killer cells in the destruction of circulating tumor emboli. J Natl Cancer Inst 65:801–809, 1980.

51. Gorelik E, Herberman RB: Radioisotope assay for evaluation of *in vivo* natural cell-mediated resistance of mice to local transplantation of tumor cells. Int J Cancer (in press).

52. Paige CJ, Figarella EF, Cuttito MJ, Cahan A, Stutman O: Natural cytotoxic cells against solid tumors in mice. II. Some characteristics of the effector cells. J Immunol 121:1827–1835, 1978.

53. Stutman O, Figarella EF, Paige CJ, Lattime EC: Natural cytotoxic (NC) cells against solid tumors in mice: general characteristics and comparison to natural killer (NK) cells. In: Natural cell-mediated immunity against tumors, Herberman RB (ed). New York: Academic Press, 1980, pp 187–229.

54. Gerson JM: Systemic and *in situ* natural killer activity in tumor-bearing mice and patients with cancer. In: Natural cell-mediated immunity against tumors, Herberman RB (ed). New York: Academic Press, 1980, pp 1047–1062.

55. Becker S, Kiessling R, Lee M, Klein G: Modulation of sensitivity to natural killer cell lysis after *in vitro* explanation of a mouse lymphoma. J Natl Cancer Inst 61:1495–1498, 1978.

56. Durdik JM, Beck BN, Henney CS: The use of lymphoma cell variants differing in their susceptibility to NK cell mediated lysis to analyze NK cell-target cell interactions. In: Natural cell-mediated immunity against tumors, Herberman RB (ed). New York: Academic Press, 1980, pp. 805–817.

57. Collins JL, Patek PQ, Cohn M: Tumorigenicity and lysis by natural killers. J Exp Med 153:89–106, 1981.

58. Kunkel LA, Welsh RM: Metabolic inhibitors render 'resistant' target cells sensitive to natural killer cell-mediated lysis. Int J Cancer 27:73–79, 1981.

59. Trinchieri G, Santoli D: Anti-viral activity induced by culturing lymphocytes with tumor-derived or virus-transformed cells. Enhancement of human natural killer cell activity by interferon and antagonistic inhibition of susceptibility of target cells to lysis. J Exp Med 147:1314–1333, 1978.

60. Welsh RM Jr, Kiessling RW: Modification of target susceptibility to activated mouse NK cells by interferon and virus infections. In: Natural cell-mediated immunity against tumors, Herberman RB (ed). New York: Academic Press, 1980, pp 963–972.

61. Herberman RB, Nunn ME, Lavrin DH: Natural cytotoxic reactivity of mouse lymphoid cells against syngeneic and allogeneic tumors. I. Distribution of reactivity and specificity. Int J Cancer 16:216–229, 1975.

62. Becker S, Klein E: Decreased 'natural killer' — NK — effect in tumor bearing mice and its relation to the immunity against oncorna virus determined cell surface antigens. Eur J Immunol 6:892–898, 1977.

63. McCoy J, Herberman R, Perlin E, Levine P, Alford C: ^{51}Cr release cellular lymphocyte cytotoxicity as a possible measure of immunological competence of cancer patients. Proc Am Assoc Cancer Res 14:107, 1973.

64. Takasugi M, Ramseyer A, Takasugi J: Decline of natural nonselective cell-mediated cytotoxicity in patients with tumor progression. Cancer Res 37:413–418, 1977.

65. Hersey P, Edwards A, McCarthy WH: Tumour-related changes in natural killer cell activity in melanoma patients. Influence of stage of disease, tumour thickness and age of patients. Int J Cancer 25:187–194, 1980.

66. Forbes JT, Greco FA, Oldham RK: Natural cell-mediated cytotoxicity in human tumor patients. In: Natural cell-mediated immunity against tumors, Herberman RB (ed). New York: Academic Press, 1980, pp 1031–1046.

67. Pross HF, Baines MG: Natural killer cells in tumour-bearing patients. In: Natural cell-mediated immunity against tumors, Herberman RB (ed). New York: Academic Press, 1980, pp 1063–1072.

68. Gerson JM, Varesio L, Herberman RB: Systemic and *in situ* natural killer and suppressor cell activities in mice bearing progressively growing murine sarcoma-virus-induced tumors.

Int J Cancer 27:243–248, 1981.
69. Vose BM: Natural killers in human cancer: Activity of tumor-infiltrating and draining node lymphocytes. In: Natural cell-mediated immunity against tumors, Herberman RB (ed). New York: Academic Press, 1980, pp 1081–1097.
70. Eremin O: NK cell activity in the blood, tumor-draining lymph nodes and primary tumours of women with mammary carcinoma. In: Natural cell-mediated immunity against tumors, Herberman RB (ed). New York: Academic Press, 1980, pp 1011–1027.
71. Allavena P, Introna M, Mangioni C, Mantovani A: Inhibition of natural killer activity by tumor-associated lymphoid cells from ascitic ovarian carcinomas. J Natl Cancer Inst (in press).
72. Brunda MJ, Herberman RB, Holden HT: Inhibition of murine natural killer cell activity by prostaglandins. J Immunol 124:2682–2687, 1980.
73. Serrate S, Herberman RB: Natural cell-mediated cytotoxicity against primary mammary tumors. Fed Proc (in press).
74. Nunn ME, Herberman RB, Holden HT: Natural cell-mediated cytotoxicity in mice against non-lymphoid tumor cells and some normal cells. Int J Cancer 20:381–387, 1977.
75. Axberg I, Gidlund M, Orn A, Pattengale P, Riesenfeld I, Stern P, Wigzell H: In: Thymus, thymic hormones and T lymphocytes, Aiuti F (ed). New York: Academic Press, 1980, pp 154–164.
76. Zarling JM, Eskra L, Borden EC, Horoszewicz J, Carter WA: Activation of human natural killer cells cytotoxic for human leukemia cells by purified interferon. J Immunol 123:63–70, 1979.
77. Vánky FT, Argov SA, Einhorn SA, Klein E: Role of alloantigens in natural killing: Allogeneic but not autologous tumor biopsy cells are sensitive for interferon-induced cytotoxicity of human blood lymphocytes. J Exp Med 151:1151–1165, 1980.
78. Mantovani A, Allavena P, Biondi A, Sessa C, Introna M: Natural killer activity in human ovarian carcinoma. In: NK cells: Fundamental aspects and role in cancer. Human cancer immunology, Vol 6, Serrou B, Herberman RB (ed). Amsterdam: North-Holland Publishing Co (in press).
79. Ortaldo JR, Oldham RK, Cannon GC, Herberman RB: Specificity of natural cytotoxic reactivity of normal human lymphocytes against a myeloid leukemia cell line. J Natl Cancer Inst 59:77–82, 1977.
80. Kiessling R, Klein E, Wigzell H: 'Natural' killer cells in the mouse. I. Cytotoxic cells with specificity for mouse Moloney leukemia cells. Specificity and distribution according to genotype. Eur J Immunol 5:112-117, 1975.
81. Becker S: Intratumor NK reactivity. In: Natural cell-mediated immunity against tumors, Herberman RB (ed). New York: Academic Press, 1980, pp 985–996.
82. Prehn RT: Immunosurveillance, regeneration and oncogenesis. Progr Exp Tumor Res 14:1–24, 1971.
83. Schwartz RS: Another look at immunologic surveillance. New Eng J Med 293:181-184, 1975.
84. Burnet FM: Cancer — a biological approach. Brit Med J 1:779–786; 841–847, 1957.
85. Thomas L: Discussion. In: Cellular and humoral aspects of the hypertensive state, Lawrence HS (ed). New York: Harper, 1959, pp 529–530.
86. Burnet FM: The concept of immunological surveillance. Progr Exp Tumor Res 13:1–27, 1970.
87. Stutman O: Immunodepression and malignancy. In: Advances in cancer research, Vol 22, Klein G, Weinhouse S, Haddow A (eds). New York: Academic Press, 1975, pp 261–422.
88. Stutman O: Chemical carcinogenesis in nude mice: Comparison between nude mice from

homozygous matings and heterozygous matings and effect of age and carcinogen dose. J Natl Cancer Inst 62:353-358, 1979.

89. Hewitt HB, Blake ER, Walder AS: A critique of the evidence for active host defence against cancer, based on personal studies of 27 murine tumours of spontaneous origin. Brit J Cancer 33:241-259, 1976.

90. Klein G, Klein E: Rejectability of virus induced tumors and non-rejectability of spontaneous tumors — a lesson in contrasts. Transpl Proc 9:1095-1104, 1977.

91. Prehn RT, Lappe MA: An immunostimulation theory of tumor development. Transpl Rev 7:26-54, 1971.

92. Goldfarb RH, Herberman RB: Characteristics of natural killer cells and possible mechanisms for their cytotoxic activity. In: Advances in inflammation research, Weissman G (ed). New York: Raven Press (in press).

93. Lotan R: Effects of vitamin A and its analogs (retinoids) on normal and neoplastic cells. Biochim Biophys Acta 605:33-37, 1980.

94. Shope TC, Kaplan J: Inhibition of the in vitro outgrowth of Epstein-Barr virus-infected lymphocytes by T_G lymphocytes. J Immunol 123:2150-2155, 1979.

95. Dent PB, Fish LA, White JF, Good RA: Chediak-Higashi syndrome. Observations on the nature of the associated malignancy. Lab Invest 15:1634-1641, 1966.

96. Roder JC, Haliotis T, Klein M, Korec S, Jett JR, Ortaldo J, Herberman RB, Katz P, Fauci AS: A new immunodeficiency disorder in humans involving NK cells. Nature 284:553-555, 1980.

97. Roder JC, Laing L, Haliotis T, Kozbor D: Genetic control of human NK function. In: NK cells: Fundamental aspects and role in cancer. Human cancer immunology, Vol 6, Serrou B, Rosenfeld C, Herberman RB (eds). Amsterdam: North-Holland Publishing Co (in press).

98. Roder JC, Lohmann-Matthes M-L, Domzig W, Wigzell H: The beige mutation in the mouse. II. Selectivity of the natural killer (NK) cell defect. J Immunol 123:2174-2181, 1979.

99. Brunda MJ, Holden HT, Herberman RB: Augmentation of natural killer cell activity of beige mice by interferon and interferon inducers. In: Natural cell-mediated immunity against tumors, Herberman RB (ed). New York: Academic Press, 1980, pp 411-415.

100. Cudkowicz G: Role of natural killer cells in natural resistance against bone marrow transplants. In: Symposium on role of natural killer cells, macrophages and antibody dependent cellular cytotoxicity in tumor rejection and as mediators of biological response modifiers activity, Chirigos MA (ed). New York: Raven Press (in press).

101. Loutit JF, Townsend KMS, Knowles JF: Tumour surveillance in beige mice. Nature 285:66, 1980.

102. Purtilo DT, De Florio D, Hutt LM, Bhawan J, Yang JPS, Otto R, Edwards W: New Engl J Med 297:1077, 1977.

103. Sullivan JL, Byron KS, Brewster FE, Purtilo DT: Deficient natural killer cell activity in X-linked lymphoproliferative syndrome. Science 210:543-545, 1980.

104. Penn I, Starzl TE: A summary of the status of de novo cancer in transplant recipients. Transpl Proc 4:719-732, 1972.

105. Lipinski M, Tursz T, Kreis H, Finale Y, Amiel JL: Dissociation of natural killer cell activity and antibody-dependent cell-mediated cytotoxicity in kidney allograft recipients receiving high-dose immunosuppressive therapy. Transplantation 29:214-218, 1980.

106. Gorelik E, Herberman RB: Inhibition of the activity of mouse NK cells by urethane. J Natl Cancer Inst 66:543-548, 1981.

107. Gorelik E, Herberman RB: Carcinogen-induced inhibition of NK activity in mice. Fed Proc 40:1093, 1981.

108. Kraskovsky G, Gorelik L, Kagan L: Abrogation of the immunosuppressive and carcinogenic action of urethan by transplantation of syngeneic bone marrow cells from normal mice. Proc Acad Sci BSSR 11:1052–1053, 1973.

109. Ehrlich R, Efrati M, Witz IP: Cytotoxicity and cytostasis mediated by splenocytes of mice subjected to chemical carcinogens and of mice bearing primary tumors. In: Natural cell-mediated immunity against tumors, Herberman RB (ed). New York: Academic Press, 1980, pp 997–1010.

110. Hochman PS, Cudkowicz G, Dausset J: Decline of natural killer cell activity in sublethally irradiated mice. J Natl Cancer Inst 61:265–268, 1978.

111. Parkinson DR, Brightman RP, Waksal SD: Altered natural killer cell biology in C57BL/6 mice after leukemogenic split-dose irradiation. J Immunol 126:1460–1464, 1981.

112. Kaplan HS, Brown MB, Paull J: Influence of bone marrow injections on involution and neoplasia of mouse thymus after systemic irradiation. J Natl Cancer Inst 14:303–316, 1953.

113. Keller R: Suppression of natural antitumor defence mechanisms by phorbol esters. Nature 282:729–731, 1979.

114. Burton RC: Alloantisera selectively reactive with NK cells: Characterization and use in defining NK cell classes. In: Natural cell-mediated immunity against tumors, Herberman RB (ed). New York: Academic Press, 1980, pp 19–35.

115. Mahoney KH, Morse SS, Morahan PS: Macrophage functions in beige (Chediak-Higashi syndrome) mice. Cancer Res 40:3934–3939, 1980.

116. Benczur M, Petrányi GG, Pálffy G, Varga M, Tálas M, Kotsy B, Földes I, Hollán SR: Dysfunction of natural killer cells in multiple sclerosis: A possible pathogenetic factor. Clin Exp Immunol 39:657–662, 1980.

117. Hoffman T: Natural killer function in systemic lupus erythematosus. Arthritis and Rheumatism 23:30–35, 1980.

118. Kiessling R, Hochman PS, Haller O, Shearer GM, Wigzell H, Cudkowicz G: Evidence for a similar or common mechanism for natural killer cell activity and resistance to hemopoietic grafts. Eur J Immunol 7:655–663, 1977.

119. Oehler JR, Herberman RB: Natural cell-mediated cytotoxicity in rats. III. Effects of immunopharmacologic treatments on natural reactivity and on reactivity augmented by polyinosinic-polycytidylic acid. Int J Cancer 21:221–229, 1978.

120. Djeu JY, Heinbaugh J, Vieira WD, Holden HT, Herberman RB: The effect of immunopharmacological agents on mouse natural cell-mediated cytotoxicity and on its augmentation by poly I:C. Immunopharmacology 1:231–244, 1979.

121. Herberman RB, Rosenberg EB, Halterman RH, McCoy JL, Leventhal BG: Cellular immune reactions to human leukemia. Natl Cancer Inst Monogr 35:259–266, 1972.

122. Introna M, Allavena P, Spreafico F, Mantovani A: Inhibition of human natural killer activity by cyclosporin A. Transplant 31:113–116, 1981.

123. Mantovani A, Luini W, Peri G, Vecchi A, Spreafico F: Effect of chemotherapeutic agents on natural cell-mediated cytotoxicity in mice. J Natl Cancer Inst 61:1255–1261, 1978.

124. Santoni A, Riccardi C, Sorci V, Herberman RB: Effects of adriamycin on the activity of mouse natural cells. J Immunol 124:2329–2335, 1980.

125. Ojo E, Wigzell H: Natural killer cells may be the only cells in normal mouse lymphoid populations endowed with cytolytic ability for antibody-coated tumor target cells. Scand J Immunol 7:297–306, 1978.

126. Landazuri MO, Silva A, Alvarez J, Herberman RB: Evidence that natural cytotoxicity and antibody dependent cellular cytotoxicity are mediated in humans by the same effector cell populations. J Immunol 123:252–258, 1979.

127. Kay HD, Bonnard GD, West WH, Herberman RB: A functional comparison of human

Fc-receptor-bearing lymphocytes active in natural cytotoxicity and antibody-dependent cellular cytotoxicity. J Immunol 118:2058–2066, 1977.

128. Ortaldo JR, Pestka S, Slease RB, Rubenstein M, Herberman RB: Augmentation of human K-cell activity with interferon. Scand J Immunol 12:365–369, 1980.

129. Djeu JY, Heinbaugh JA, Holden HT, Herberman RB: Augmentation of mouse natural killer cell activity by interferon and interferon inducers. J Immunol 122:175–181, 1979.

130. Gidlund M. Örn A, Wigzell H, Senik A, Gresser I: Enhanced NK cell activity in mice injected with interferon and interferon inducers. Nature 223:259–261, 1978.

131. Herberman RB, Ortaldo JR, Bonnard GD: Augmentation by interferon of human natural and antibody-dependent cell-mediated cytotoxicity. Nature 277:221–223, 1979.

132. Santoli D, Trinchieri G, Koprowski H: Cell-mediated cytotoxicity against virus-infected target cells in humans. II. Interferon induction and activation of natural killer cells. J Immunol 121:532–538, 1978.

133. Timonen T, Ortaldo JR, Herberman RB: Characteristics of human large granular lymphocytes and relationship to natural killer and K cells. J Exp Med 153:569–582, 1981.

134. Herberman RB, Ortaldo JR, Djeu JY, Holden HT, Jett J, Lang NP, Pestka S: Role of interferon in regulation of cytotoxicity by natural killer cells and macrophages. Ann NY Acad Sci 350:63–71, 1980.

135. Herberman RB, Ortaldo JR, Rubinstein M, Pestka S: Augmentation of natural and antibody-dependent cell-mediated cytotoxicity by pure human leukocyte interferon. J Clin Immunol (in press).

136. Herberman RB, Brunda MJ, Cannon GB, Djeu JY, Nunn-Hargrove ME, Jett JR, Ortaldo JR, Reynolds C, Riccardi C, Santoni A: Augmentation of natural killer (NK) cell activity by interferon-inducers. In: Augmenting agents in cancer therapy. Current status and future prospects, Hersh E, Mastrangelo M (eds). New York: Raven Press (in press).

137. Santoni A, Riccardi C, Barlozzari T, Herberman RB: Inhibition as well as augmentation of mouse NK activity by pyran copolymer and adriamycin. In: Natural cell-mediated immunity against tumors, Herberman RB (ed). New York: Academic Press, 1980, pp 753–763.

138. Strausser HR, Humes JL: Prostaglandin synthesis inhibition: effect on bone changes and sarcoma tumor induction in BALB/c mice. Int J Cancer 15:724–730, 1975.

139. Lynch NR, Castes M. Astoin M, Salomon JC: Mechanism of inhibition of tumour growth by aspirin and indomethacin. Brit J Cancer 38:503–512, 1978.

140. Lupulescu A: Enhancement of carcinogenesis by prostaglandins. Nature 272:634–636, 1978.

141. Plescia OJ, Smith AH, Grinwich K: Subversion of immune system by tumor cells and role of prostaglandins. Proc Natl Acad Sci 72:1848–1851, 1975.

142. Lynch NR, Salomon JC: Tumor growth inhibition and potentiation of immunotherapy by indomethacin in mice. J Natl Cancer Inst 62:117–125, 1979.

2. Clonal Evolution and Childhood Tumors

PETER C. NOWELL and GLORIA B. BALABAN

1. INTRODUCTION

Many of the clinical and biological characteristics of tumor development appear to fit with the view that most neoplasms are unicellular in origin (i.e., 'clones') and that tumor progression results from 'clonal evolution', the sequential appearance within unstable neoplastic clones of subpopulations which are more and more genetically aberrant. These concepts, and the suggested underlying mechanisms, will be reviewed briefly, along with some of the supporting evidence. Although relatively few data are available from tumors occurring in the pediatric age group, some examples from both hematopoietic and nonhematopoietic neoplasms will be summarized. The findings support the general applicability of these concepts to pediatric neoplasms, but certain special characteristics of this age group require consideration, and these will be discussed from the standpoint of both their theoretical and practical implications.

2. THE CLONAL EVOLUTION HYPOTHESIS

There is increasing evidence from cytogenetic, biochemical, and immunological studies that most tumors are of unicellular origin. A simplified formulation would suggest that a carcinogen (radiation, chemical, virus) interacts with the genome of a single cell to confer on that cell a heritable selective growth advantage. When that cell divides, its progeny escape to some degree from local growth regulation and begin clonal expansion as a neoplasm.

Studies with modern cytogenetic banding techniques have supported this model by demonstrating that abnormalities are often the same throughout all the cells of a given tumor. Where there is a spectrum of cytogenetic

G. B. Humphrey et al. (eds.), Pancreatic Tumors in Children.
© 1982 Martinus Nijhoff Publishers, The Hague / Boston / London. ISBN-13:978-94-009-7617-7

changes, these are often demonstrably related. Even in highly malignant solid neoplasms with much karyotypic variation, characteristic marker chromosomes, recognizable in all cells of a given tumor, indicate that the entire neoplastic population is derived from a single cell of origin [1, 2].

Biochemical studies of the distribution of the enzyme G6PD in many tumors [3], and immunological data on the monoclonal characteristics of the immunoglobulin produced by a number of lymphoproliferative neoplasms also support this clonal concept. It should be stressed that the term 'clone' is being used here only to indicate the unicellular origin of the tumor and not homogeneity of the neoplastic population. Since a malignancy in its later stages, through somatic mutation, may often come to consist of a large number of genetically different subpopulations derived from the original clone, it is not surprising that many tumors prove heterogeneous for whatever phenotypic characteristic is being examined [4]. Also, it should be noted that this clonal hypothesis does not rule out the possibility that application of a carcinogen to an organ or to an area of skin can produce many potentially neoplastic cells; it simply indicates that as a tumor evolves from such an area, the progeny of one or, at most, a very few cells ultimately overgrow the site and account for the macroscopic neoplasm.

There are a few exceptions to this generalization of clonal origin, including some tumors in the pediatric age group. The exceptions are primarily tumors of viral etiology (for example, condylomata acuminata) where there has possibly been infection of adjacent cells, or they are neoplasms with a strong hereditary component (such as neurofibromatosis) where a familial gene defect presumably involves every cell and greatly increases its susceptibility to neoplastic change [5, 6].

The vast majority of neoplasms, however, appear to be 'clonal', as defined, with the tumor arising from the progeny of a single cell which has acquired a heritable selective growth advantage through interaction with a carcinogen. The exact nature of this interaction, and the key alteration in the neoplastic cell, remains uncertain, despite extensive speculation and search. Although the acquired selective growth advantage within the neoplastic clone acts like a somatic mutation, this initial event apparently need not always involve an irreversible alteration in the structure or function of the genome.

In some instances, the probability of this critical somatic change may be increased by an inherited gene or chromosome defect in all the cells of the individual. For example, certain tumors (e.g., retinoblastoma and neuroblastoma) exist in hereditary as well as nonhereditary form, with the hereditary cases occurring at an earlier age, and often as multiple tumors. Knudson [7] attempted to explain these observations with a 'two hit' model which suggests that a cell requires two genetic alterations to become neo-

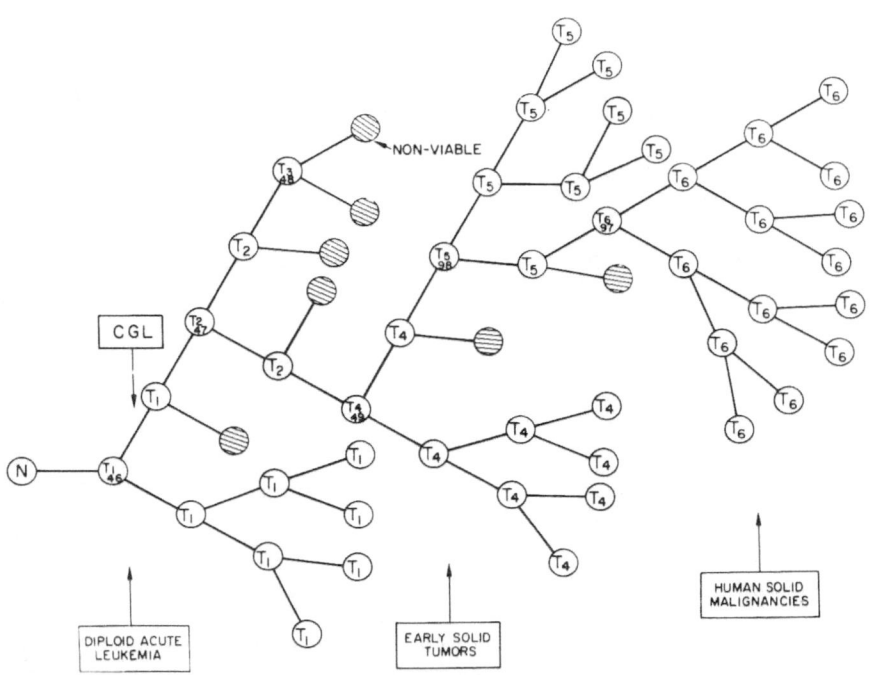

Figure 1. Model of clonal evolution in neoplasia. Carcinogen-induced change in progenitor normal cell (N) produces a diploid tumor cell (T_1, 46 chromosomes), with growth advantage permitting clonal expansion to begin. Genetic instability of T_1 cells leads to production of variants (illustrated by changes in chromosome number, T_2 to T_6). Most variants die, due to metabolic or immunologic disadvantage (hatched circles); occasionally one has an additional selective advantage (for example, T_2, 47 chromosomes), and its progeny become the predominant subpopulation until an even more favorable variant appears (for example, T_4). The step-wise sequence in each tumor differs (being partially determined by environmental pressures on selection), and results in a different, aneuploid karyotype predominating in each fully developed malignancy (T_6). Earlier subpopulations (for example, T_1, T_4, T_5) may persist sufficiently to contribute to heterogeneity within the advanced tumor. Biological characteristics of tumor progression (e.g., morphological and metabolic loss of differentiation, invasion and metastasis, resistance to therapy) parallel the stages of genetic evolution. Human tumors with minimal chromosome change (diploid acute leukemia, chronic granulocytic leukemia) are considered to be early in clonal evolution; adult cancers, typically highly aneuploid, are viewed as late in the developmental process (from Nowell [13]).

plastic. In hereditary cases, all cells would have an initial mutation as an inherited gene defect, and so would only have to acquire one additional change to become neoplastic [7, 8], greatly increasing this probability. This hereditary component of tumorigenesis is of major importance in some pediatric neoplasms and will be discussed later in more detail.

28

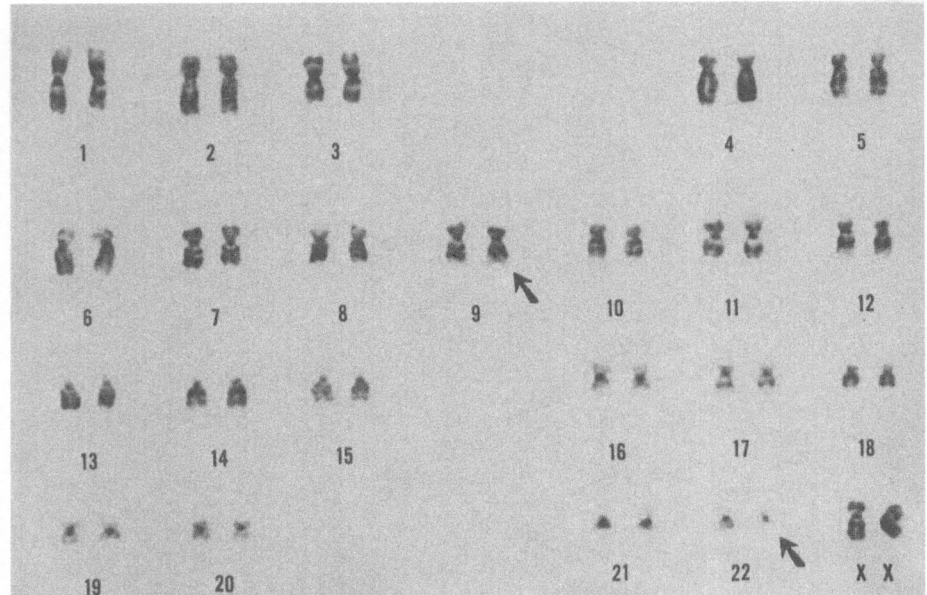

Figure 2. Banded karyotype from a patient with chronic granulocytic leukemia (CGL) in the early, indolent stage. The typical translocation from chromosome 22 to chromosome 9 (arrows), producing the Philadelphia chromosome (22 q⁻), was present in the cells of the neoplastic clone.

Whatever the nature of the initial cellular alteration, it permits the neoplastic population to begin to expand, and then the second component of the clonal evolution hypothesis becomes important. It has been suggested by a number of workers [9–13] that the clinical and biological events described as 'tumor progression' represent the effects of genetic instability in the neoplastic cells, and the sequential selection of variant subpopulations produced as a result of that instability. A model describing this concept is illustrated in Figure 1. In this formulation of clonal evolution, most variants arising in the tumor cell population do not survive; but those few mutants which have a selective growth advantage expand to become predominant subpopulations within the neoplasm and demonstrate the characteristics which we recognize as tumor progression (e.g., invasion and metastasis, increased growth rate, loss of differentiation). The continued presence of multiple subpopulations within the tumor, as illustrated in Figure 1, provides the basis for the heterogeneity which is typically observed [4].

2.1. Evidence that Clonal Evolution Underlies Tumor Progression

Chromosome studies have provided most of the data which support the

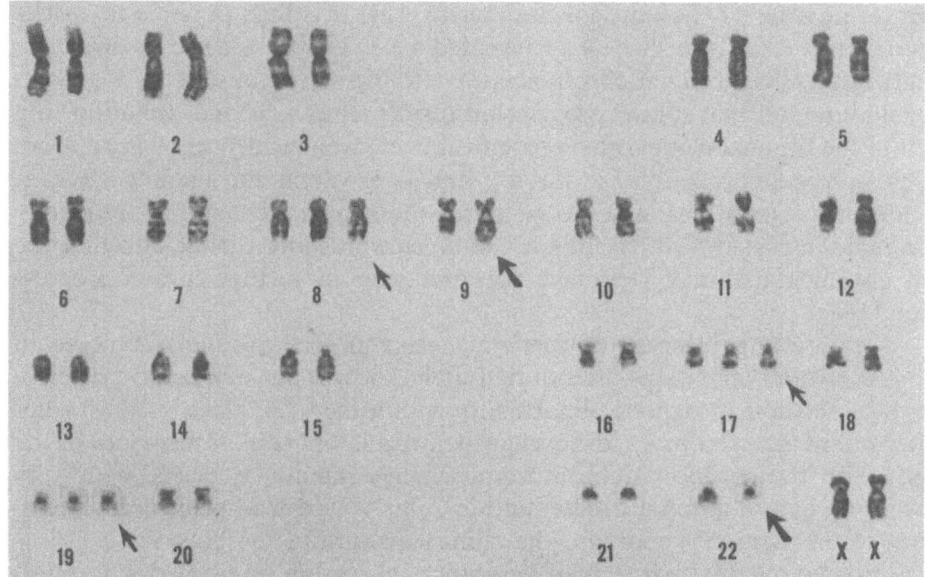

Figure 3. Banded karyotype from a patient with CGL in the terminal accelerated phase. In addition to the 9;22 translocation, there are three extra chromosomes (8, 17, and 19). Clinical progression of the disease was associated with overgrowth of the original Ph-positive neoplastic cells by a subclone with these additional cytogenetic changes.

clonal evolution concept. In general, advanced malignancies show more extensive chromosomal aberrations than earlier stages of neoplasia [2, 14]. In a few instances, it has been possible to follow, over time, the progression of a human neoplasm to more 'malignant' characteristics and to demonstrate an association with the emergence of new predominant subpopulations of tumor cells having additional genetic alterations, recognizable cytogenetically.

This phenomenon has been best documented in chronic granulocytic leukemia (CGL), where both the early and late stages are usually accompanied by chromosomal abnormalities. In the early, indolent stage of typical CGL in the adult (and in the so-called 'adult-type' disease in children), the neoplastic cells nearly always contain the Philadelphia chromosome (a translocation from the long arm of chromosome 22, usually to the long arm of chromosome 9) as the only cytogenetic change (Figure 2). After several years, when the accelerated phase or 'blast crisis' occurs, a subpopulation of cells with karyotypic abnormalities in addition to the Philadelphia (Ph) chromosome often is predominant (Figure 3). These additional changes are not consistent from case to case, but frequently involve one or more of several specific alterations (a second Ph, an isochromosome for the long arm of number 17, trisomy for number 8) [15]. It is thus possible to speculate that in CGL the disease is initiated by a visible genetic change in a marrow stem cell (the Ph chromosome), altering its response to local growth regulation, and that tumor progression results from a second mutation in a cell of the original clone, often recognizable cytogenetically, allowing a more aggressive subpopulation to develop and overwhelm the patient. (Recent evidence suggests that in some instances the neoplastic clone in CGL may originate in a stem cell having no visible chromosome change and that the Ph chromosome may represent the first step in further tumor progression [16].)

As with all neoplasms, the specific genes and gene products involved in both early and late stages are not definitely known, but one could postulate that the second cytogenetic abnormality within the CGL clone might further alter membrane receptors for local growth regulators so that nearly all of the cells with the additional chromosome change remain as blasts, with very few undergoing terminal differentiation. This would lead to a rapid expansion of the stem cell pool and the clinical picture of the blast crisis.

Similar sequential patterns of karyotypic alteration associated with clinical progression have been reported in other human leukemic and preleukemic disorders [2, 14], but many cases do not follow the protracted time course necessary for repeated investigations. We have recently followed for five years a patient with chronic T cell leukemia who ultimately developed a rapidly growing diffuse histiocytic lymphoma, a sequence recognized as Richter's syndrome. Abnormal marker chromosomes in the cells of the leukemia were also present in the lymphoma, indicating its derivation from the original neoplasm [17].

There are also some chromosomal data from experimental animals which support the concept of clonal evolution underlying tumor progression. In a number of primary sarcomas induced in mice and rats by the Rous virus, the karyotype was initially normal [18, 19]. Serial biopsies of individual tumors as they gradually acquired more malignant properties (e.g., increased growth rate, reduced collagen production) revealed the sequential appearance of new sublines, identified cytogenetically, overgrowing and replacing the original diploid tumor cells. These karyotypic alterations apparently provided selective growth advantages over earlier populations within the neoplasm.

The various findings cited above indicate that, through cytogenetic techniques, the sequential appearance of more and more genetically aberrant subpopulations has been demonstrable in a number of human and animal tumors, paralleling new and more aggressive characteristics of the neoplastic cells, and thus supporting the concept of tumor progression illustrated in Figure 1.

2.2. Genetic Lability of Tumor Cells

Before considering clinical implications of these observations, as well as pediatric tumors and their special characteristics, one important aspect of the general hypothesis just discussed needs more detailed review: the genetic instability of neoplastic cells which is presumed to underlie clonal evolution. What is the evidence that tumor cell populations are genetically unstable, and if so, what might be the causative mechanisms?

When tumors are examined histologically, one is often struck by the presence of obvious mitotic abnormalities. In fact, such observations led workers such as Boveri and Von Hansemann [20, 21] to the earliest theories concerning an important role of chromosomal alterations in the development of cancer. Histologic studies also suggest that the genetic instability represented by mitotic abnormalities may become more pronounced as a neoplasm evolves. In advanced malignancies, a wide range of mitotic variants are commonly observed with each cell generation, as compared to relatively few in early benign lesions [22].

Experimental data which also suggest that tumor cell populations are more genetically labile than comparable normal cells are being reported with increased frequency. Both *in vivo* and *in vitro*, there is evidence that neoplastic cells may be more susceptible to chromosome breakage, nondisjunction and ploidy changes, sister chromatid exchange (SCE), and other genetic alterations than comparable normal cells [23–28]. There are even limited experimental data indicating that this enhanced mutability increases with tumor progression.

A variety of mechanisms could account for this apparent increased mutability of tumor cell populations, providing the basis for clonal evolution and tumor progression. The possibilities suggested below are by no means mutually exclusive, and at various stages of tumor development and in different neoplasms, different mechanisms could operate.

2.2.1. Inherited Defects. In a small segment of the population, and particularly in the pediatric age group, increased genetic instability in neoplastic cells may not result from an acquired alteration, but rather reflect an inherited gene defect present in all cells of the body. Individuals with the so-called 'chromosome breakage syndromes' (Bloom's syndrome, Fanconi's anemia, ataxia-telangiectasia, xeroderma pigmentosum) [29–31], apparently have an inherited defect in DNA repair, or in some other aspect of DNA 'housekeeping', although the details have not been completely worked out in all instances. As a somewhat oversimplified generalization, it can be suggested that genetic lability in the patient's cells resulting from the inherited gene defect leads to chromosome aberrations, cytogenetically abnormal

clones, and ultimately the increased incidence of neoplasia which character-
izes these syndromes.

It is possible that inherited gene defects with similar effects may be present in individuals without recognizable clinical syndromes. There have
been children described, for instance, with unexplained familial disorders of
blood formation who do not fit one of the recognized chromosome breakage
diseases [32, 33]. These children may demonstrate cytogenetically abnormal
clones among circulating lymphocytes or in the bone marrow, and some
ultimately progress to leukemia. It has not yet been demonstrated that such
patients carry gene defects influencing karyotypic stability, but the parallels
with known chromosome breakage syndromes suggest that this may be the
case.

It has also been recognized that the cells of individuals with constitutional
chromosome abnormalities, in particular Down's syndrome, show evidence
of increased susceptibility to cytogenetic damage and rearrangement when
exposed to clastogenic agents *in vitro* [34]. It is not clear whether the specific
chromosomal alteration in the patient's cells has, itself, a destabilizing
effect, or whether both the constitutional abnormality and the increased
fragility reflect an inherited defect in chromosomal stability analogous to
that discussed in the preceding paragraphs. In at least some families, the
latter possibility seems supported by the presence of different constitutional
chromosome alterations in family members as well as a general familial
increase in cancer incidence [35, 36].

2.2.2. Acquired Defects. For the vast majority of patients with cancer, it is
assumed that there is no constitutional abnormality in genetic stability, and
that the increased lability within the neoplastic clone is the result of an
acquired alteration. Many kinds of acquired defects have been suggested by
various workers, with some supporting evidence in studies of different
tumors.

Single gene mutations of various types could destabilize the genome. Such
'mutator genes' might result in abnormalities in DNA repair similar to
those in the chromosome breakage syndromes; abnormalities in the DNA
synthetic apparatus, increasing the utilization of more error-prone path-
ways; or even instability of the mitotic spindle resulting in abnormalities of
the mitotic process. There are reports consistent with the action of each of
these various types of mutator genes in certain neoplastic cell populations [9, 37, 38].

In addition to such single gene lesions, one can also postulate that chromosomal alterations, once established within the tumor cell population,
may themselves contribute to the continuing and perhaps increasing genetic
instability within the neoplastic cells. Aneuploidy, for instance, could result

from one of the mutagenic mutations suggested in the preceding paragraph, and so might appear during evolution of the tumor. Once present, it could contribute to the production of further genetic errors [34].

Even balanced translocations in a neoplastic cell might cause differential gene expression due to 'position effect'. For instance, the portion of chromosome 8 translocated onto chromosome 14 in Burkitt's lymphoma shows a color shift when stained with acridine orange. It has been suggested that this color shift may reflect a change from inactive heterochromatin to active euchromatin [39]. Recently, the related idea of 'transposable elements' has been reintroduced as a possible important consideration in neoplasia [40, 41]. In this concept, certain DNA segments may move about within the genome and exert various kinds of destabilizing effects on other segments, adjacent to their sites of insertion.

Several additional types of chromosome alterations, recognizable in tumor cells, might also increase genetic instability in the neoplastic clone as well as having specific immediate effects in terms of alterations in gene products. For instance, the phenomenon of homogeneously staining regions (HSR) and related double minutes (DMs) could have such a dual effect. These novel chromosome abnormalities are largely confined to tumor cells. The HSR is a long, unbanded region of excess DNA in a chromosome, which apparently represents an area of gene amplification. The increased gene product from this site may have an important role in the growth of certain neoplasms [42]. Double minutes are small paired chromatin bodies which lack centromeres. Some may therefore be lost at each cell division. If, as has been suggested, an HSR can break down into separate DMs which can be lost from the cell, this mechanism could contribute to genetic instability in the system (Figure 4) [43].

Finally, it has been suggested that somatic exchanges between chromatids of homologous chromosomes may be important in tumor development, by generating homozygosity of critical recessive genes [44]. If a mutagenic mutation in a neoplastic clone resulted in an increased frequency of such chromatid exchanges, the probability of further significant genetic alterations within the population might thus be enhanced [45].

These various considerations indicate that a number of kinds of acquired specific mutations and chromosomal alterations may underlie the observed genetic lability in different tumor cell populations, operating through various forms of gene duplication, deletion, position effects, and imbalance. There is little firm evidence to suggest the relative importance of different types of alterations, although Cairns [46] has recently suggested that gross chromosomal lesions may be of greater importance in human neoplasia than point mutations.

It should be recognized that various types of genetic change could occur at

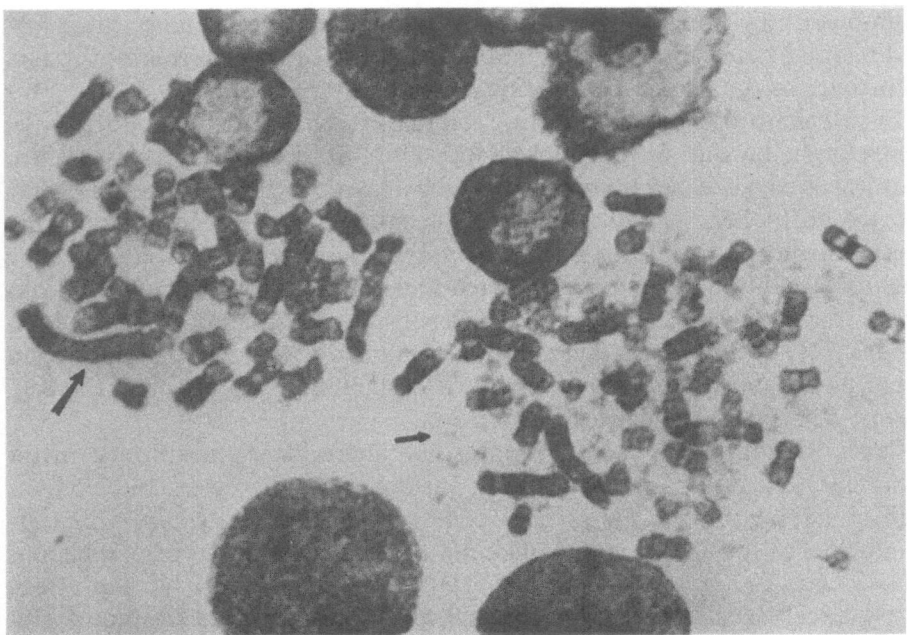

Figure 4. Adjacent metaphases from human neuroblastoma cell line (CHP-126), showing two classes of cells: one with homogeneously staining region (HSR) (large arrow) and one with double minutes (DMs) (small arrow). It is postulated that HSR may break down into DMs, leading to changes in the neoplastic characteristics of the cell.

different times during tumor development, even within the same neoplasm. We have already noted that chromosomal alterations might result from a gene mutation acquired earlier, and then, in turn, contribute to a cascade of increasing instability. It is also worth pointing out that in some instances the acquired mutagenic mutation might actually occur *before* the cell which ultimately initiates a neoplastic clone acquires a permanent selective growth advantage and so qualifies as 'neoplastic' in our working definition.

2.2.3. Extracellular Factors. In addition to these inherited and acquired mechanisms which may underline genetic instability in different neoplasms, it is also possible that extracellular factors may contribute to the sequential mutational events involved in clonal evolution. If, for instance, an oncogenic virus is the causative agent, its incorporation into the genome of the cell may not only trigger the initial transformation event, but could also have a continuing destabilizing effect on adjacent segments of the host cell genome. Some theories of viral oncogenesis, such as Temin's 'provirus' concept [47], have envisioned viral elements as functioning, in some respects, like the 'transposable elements' described above.

Similarly, the continued presence of a long-lived carcinogenic chemical or radioisotope in an individual, or repeated doses of such clastogenic materials through occupational or other exposure, could also result in sequential mutations within the tumor. Even the mutagenic therapeutic agents used in cancer treatment (radiation, chemotherapy) might contribute significantly in this way to later stages of clonal evolution and tumor progression in some patients, as well as to the induction of a second neoplasm, as will be discussed later.

2.3. Clinical Implications of the Clonal Evolution Hypothesis

The general view of tumor development which has been presented is somewhat discouraging from the standpoint of clinical control of cancer. The hope for many years has been to find a consistent metabolic alteration in tumor cells which could be exploited therapeutically. It seems increasingly likely that if such a common molecular change does occur as the first step in many neoplasms, it may initially represent only a relatively minor quantitative change in a critical gene product. Furthermore, its identification in a tumor is made extremely difficult by the many evolutionary steps, indicated in Figure 1, between the initial change and the fully developed malignancy as one sees it clinically.

These sequential stages are not only multiple, but also to some degree random, reflecting the particular environmental pressures that influence the development of each tumor. Under these circumstances, one may ultimately have to consider each advanced malignancy as an individual therapeutic problem. In addition, the definite handicap to the therapist which the genetic lability of the tumor cell population will impose must still be recognized. The same capacity for variation and selection which permitted the evolution of a malignant population from the original aberrant cell also provides the opportunity for the tumor to adapt successfully to whatever treatment the physician may devise. Special aspects of these problems as they apply to pediatric neoplasms will be considered in the sections which follow.

3. CLONAL EVOLUTION IN PEDIATRIC TUMORS

A general model of tumor development and some of the evidence on which it is based have been presented. We will now consider this model in relation to a number of tumors of childhood: leukemia, lymphoma, and nonhematopoietic malignancy.

3.1. Leukemia

Cytogenetic studies of the acute leukemias of childhood have provided evidence on the clonal nature of these disorders, and in some instances provided support for the view that clonal evolution is associated with tumor progression. Approximately half the cases of childhood leukemia are chromosomally abnormal, and several studies indicate that these tumors are less responsive to therapy than those with a normal karyotype [48, 49], presumably because the former cases are further advanced in clonal evolution (see Figure 1). In a few instances, sequential studies of individual patients have been done, and when relapse involved a new subline with additional chromosome changes, the prognosis for successful treatment was particularly poor [48]. Apparently, as in bacteria, such a subline often represents a drug-resistant mutant, and it is possible that cytogenetic monitoring for the early appearance of these cells might permit alternative therapy before the new subpopulation predominates.

Similar evolutionary patterns have also been observed in Ph-positive chronic granulocytic leukemia in childhood. We have studied several children in the later stages of CGL in whom the frequency of blasts in the circulation and the aggressiveness of the disease correlated with the proportion of cells containing chromosome alterations in addition to the Philadelphia chromosome. As with the acute leukemias, cytogenetic monitoring of these subpopulations, some of which may have lymphoid characteristics [15], may occasionally assist the physician in determining the most appropriate therapy at different times.

Of particular interest are the rare cases of chronic T cell leukemia arising in children with ataxia-telangiectasia (AT). These provide some of the best documented examples of clonal evolution in human neoplasia, with some understanding of the underlying genetic instability. There are several reports of families with AT in whom nonneoplastic lymphocyte clones, identified by chromosome abnormalities, have been present in the blood of one or more children over several years. In some instances, these clones have shown little indication of continued expansion, and in other cases there has been eventual progression to T cell leukemia [50–52]. A frequent cytogenetic abnormality in these clones has been a translocation involving various sites in the long arm of chromosome 14 (14q). During the indolent phase, a rearrangement has been more commonly noted in the proximal portion of 14q (band q12); while in the aggressive phase, there has usually been involvement of the terminal portion (band q24–32). This latter abnormality has been observed in a variety of lymphoid neoplasms, and it has been suggested as the site of a specific gene, perhaps involving immunoglobulin synthesis, which when altered can somehow provide a marked selective growth advantage for lymphoid cells [11, 53].

In these patients with AT, one can suggest that genetic instability in the system would result from the inherited defect in DNA repair, and the associated immune dysfunction in these individuals could contribute to unbalanced proliferation of various lymphoid subsets. The combination of instability and increased proliferation could lead to chromosomal rearrangements, clones with various degrees of selective advantage, and ultimately involvement of the terminal portion of 14q (with or without additional cytogenetic changes) resulting in a clone expanding rapidly enough to be considered a true neoplasm [32]. Interestingly, a similar sequence of events has been described in a patient with Fanconi's anemia (FA) [53].

3.2. Lymphoma

As with the leukemias, cytogenetic data, as well as immunological marker studies, indicate the clonal nature of lymphomas occurring in the pediatric age group [50, 51, 52]. Studies of the Burkitt tumor have been of particular interest, and suggest a sequence of events similar to that described for the leukemias arising in AT patients. The Burkitt lymphoma is frequently characterized by a translocation from the long arm of chromosome 8 to the long arm of chromosome 14 (band q24–32). In a formulation similar to that suggested by Klein [11], it has been suggested that infection with the Epstein-Barr virus could be the source of genetic instability in this lymphoid population. Malarial infection could represent a nonspecific stimulus for the cells to proliferate; and the combination of instability and proliferation could result in an occasional cell acquiring the specific translocation from 8q to the terminal portion of 14q which leads to emergence of a frankly neoplastic clone.

Such a postulated sequence of events for AT and for the Burkitt lymphoma may be oversimplified, but it does permit various phenomena apparently of importance in tumor development to be fitted into earlier concepts of 'initiation' and 'promotion' [55, 56]. In this view, characteristics of the 'initiated' cell could include both genetic instability and/or heritable growth advantage (without necessarily any visible chromosome change), and 'promotion' would be the proliferative stimulus which allows the effects of both of these characteristics to be expressed in an actively dividing population, resulting in the acquisition of further significant genetic alterations and more aggressive biological behavior.

3.3. Nonhematopoietic Malignancies

Only limited data are available on the clonal nature of nonhematopoietic solid malignancies in children, and even less on the relationship of clonal evolution to clinical and biological progression. The relative rarity of the pediatric tumors has made it even more difficult than in adults to obtain cytogenetic studies in solid malignancies, particularly of a sequential nature. The few cytogenetic observations with respect to evolution tend to support the clonal concept. Orye and Delbeke [57] reported chromosome data in five cases of CNS tumors or retinoblastomas in children. The findings indicated a clonal pattern of growth in each instance, and the presence of multiple related sublines, identifiable cytogenetically, was interpreted by the authors as evidence of clonal evolution having occurred within the neoplasms.

Studies of HSRs and DMs in cell lines established from neuroblastomas have suggested the possibility of an unusual mechanism for clonal evolution in these pediatric tumors. Balaban-Malenbaum and Gilbert [58], as noted above, reported indirect evidence that HSRs in cultured cells can break down into separate DMs which are ultimately lost from the cell (Figure 4). Recent data suggest that the same phenomenon may occur *in vivo* [59]. In addition to contributing to genetic instability in neuroblastoma populations, leading to further clonal evolution, it is also theoretically possible that the breakdown of an HSR could result in reconstitution of a normal chromosome and reduction in malignant characteristics within a given cell [43]. Unfortunately, unless such a change occurred in most cells of a tumor, it would have little effect on growth *in vivo*.

Two other solid malignancies of childhood, retinoblastoma and Wilms' tumor, have provided important data relevant to genetic alterations in human neoplasia. Best documented is the syndrome in children born with a deletion of a portion of the long arm of chromosome 13, characterized by mental retardation, various physical defects, and a high incidence of retinoblastoma [8]. Special banding studies [60], as well as our recent data on retinoblastoma cells from individuals with a normal constitutional karyotype [61, 62], have provided strong evidence of a particular location in 13q (band q14) as being the site of a gene associated with the development of this neoplasm. Although this locus obviously plays some key role in allowing retinal cells to escape from growth control (and perhaps cells in other tissues as well), it is not clear whether this action is mediated through a specific gene product or through a destabilizing effect of this abnormality on adjacent segments of the genome, increasing the probability of various kinds of mutational events.

A similar circumstance has been observed in several cases of Wilms' tumor associated with aniridia, where a constitutional deletion in one band of the short arm of chromosome 11 has been demonstrated, pointing to this locus as being important in the etiology of the tumor [63]. These findings indicate that constitutional cytogenetic abnormalities may occasionally help to indicate the location of genes specific for particular human solid malignancies, but it appears that, at least with present techniques, such associations will be very rare.

In general, the cytogenetic data on nonhematopoietic pediatric malignancies have, thus, provided more information concerning specific gene loci relevant to cancer, than on the role of clonal evolution in the development of these neoplasms. Although the limited findings to date are consistent with the general clonal evolution hypothesis, the data both on specific chromosome abnormalities and on changes in cytogenetic patterns over time are too fragmentary to be of prognostic value at present.

3.4. Special Characteristics of Pediatric Tumors Relevant to Clonal Evolution

There are two aspects of pediatric neoplasia which warrant brief additional discussion. One is somewhat encouraging from a clinical standpoint, and the other more discouraging. The encouraging observation is the occasional 'spontaneous' cure of certain pediatric malignancies (e.g., neuroblastoma, teratocarcinoma), suggesting the possibility of reversing the malignant state. These phenomena are not fully understood, but one can speculate that a number of these childhood neoplasms can be considered, to some degree, 'embryonic rests' in an actively proliferating stage of development, and presumably still somewhat responsive to normal differentiating influences [64–67]. Because of their 'embryonic' state these cells may not require as extensive genetic alteration to acquire 'malignant' characteristics as in adults, and so may be earlier in clonal evolution (the left side of Figure 1) than most adult cancers. There is limited evidence that such cells can be manipulated *in vitro* and *in vivo* to differentiate, through such procedures as the exposure of neuroblastoma cells to nerve growth factor in culture [68] or the transplantation of a teratocarcinoma cell into an early blastocyst [69].

When such tumors, as well as some of the childhood leukemias, retain a diploid or near-diploid karyotype, the possibility of altering the environment *in vivo* to force them into normal patterns of controlled differentiation seem more hopeful than for the common adult malignancies indicated on the right in Figure 1, which are typically highly aneuploid. At present, we remain largely ignorant of both the stimulatory growth factors (e.g., nerve growth factor, epidermal growth factor) and inhibitory agents (e.g., chalones) which normally regulate the balance between proliferation and differentiation at the local level. Based on the limited evidence to date, however, it seems that certain pediatric tumors may be among the best candidates for attempts to reverse the malignant phenotype.

On the negative side, with respect to childhood neoplasms, is the observation already discussed, that a significant number of these tumors may be arising in individuals with constitutional deficiencies in genetic stability. In some instances, these may involve the recognized chromosome breakage syndromes, but other types of constitutional cytogenetic anomalies and genetic instability may be occurring as an inherited defect in a greater proportion of the population than is currently recognized. As already noted, such a defect can increase the probability both of an initial neoplastic change in a cell and of subsequent clonal evolution in the resultant neoplasm, with clinical progression to more malignant characteristics. Inherited defects in DNA repair or some other aspect of DNA 'housekeeping' may make every cell in the body more susceptible to neoplastic transformation by various carcinogenic agents, including viruses, and the immune deficiencies associated with many of these genetic disorders may also contribute to increased tumor incidence [33]. Not only will these individuals have an enhanced probability for multiple tumors as well as for neoplasms of multicellular origin, but they will also be more susceptible to the induction of secondary tumors when their first neoplasms are treated by mutagenic agents such as radiation or chemotherapy [69].

Both the possible reversibility of certain childhood tumors and the increased genetic lability in some pediatric cancer patients provide special opportunities to investigate critical aspects of tumor development in man. From such studies may eventually come better understanding of these processes and opportunities for improved prevention and control.

4. SUMMARY

1. There is increasing evidence that most tumors, including those in the pediatric age group, are clones (i.e., unicellular in origin); and that the clinical and biological phenomena of tumor progression and heterogeneity result from 'clonal evolution', genetic variation within the original clone allowing sequential selection of more aggressive subpopulations over time.

2. Available evidence also indicates that most tumor cell populations are, to some degree, more genetically unstable than comparable normal cells. This lability provides the basis for clonal evolution and may result from inherited gene defects, or from acquired alterations in the neoplastic cells.

3. Sequential genetic changes in neoplastic clones may be recognizable cytogenetically. Chromosome studies, as well as other approaches, are providing evidence for clonal evolution in human tumors, and also beginning to elucidate some of the underlying mechanisms.

4. Pediatric studies are of particular interest because they include neoplasms particularly susceptible to normal growth regulators as well as models of genetic instability in recognized tumor-associated syndromes.

5. In a few instances, particularly involving hematopoietic neoplasms, cytogenetic evidence of specific alterations, as well as of the stage of clonal evolution, may provide useful diagnostic and prognostic information for the pediatric oncologist and hematologist.

REFERENCES

1. Harnden D: The relationship between induced chromosome aberrations and chromosome abnormality in tumor cells. In: Human Genetics, Armendares S, Lisker R (eds). Amsterdam: Excerpta Medica, 1977, pp 355–366.
2. Nowell P: Cytogenetics. In: Cancer: A Comprehensive Treatise, Vol I, Etiology, Becker F (ed). New York: Plenum, 1982, pp 3–46.
3. Fialkow P: Clonal origin of human tumors. Ann Rev Med 30:135–143, 1979.
4. Heppner GH, Shapiro WR, Rankin JK: Tumor heterogeneity. In: Pediatric Oncology, Vol 1, Humphrey GB, Dehner LP, Grindey GB, Acton RT (eds). The Hague: Martinus Nijhoff, 1981, pp 99–116.
5. Linder D, Gartler SM: Glocuse-6-phosphate dehydrogenase mosaicism: utilization as a cell marker in the study of leiomyomas. Science 150:67–69, 1965.
6. Friedman JM, Fialkow P: Viral 'tumorigenesis' in man: cell markers in *condylomata acuminata*. Int J Cancer 17:57–61, 1976.
7. Knudson AG: Mutation and cancer: statistical study of retinoblastoma. Proc Nat Acad Sci USA 68:820–823, 1971.
8. Knudson A, Meadows A, Nichols W, Hill R: Chromosomal deletion and retinoblastoma. N Eng J Med 295:1120–1123, 1976.
9. Cairns J: Mutation, selection, and the natural history of cancer. Nature 255:197–200, 1975.
10. De Grouchy J, De Nava C: A chromosomal theory of carcinogenesis. Ann Int Med 69:381–391, 1968.
11. Klein G: Lymphoma development in mice and humans: diversity of initiation is followed by convergent cytogenetic evolution. Proc Natl Acad Sci USA 76:2442–2446, 1979.
12. Makino S: Further evidence favoring the concept of the stem cell in ascites tumors of rats. Ann NY Acad Sci 64:818–823, 1956.
13. Nowell P: The clonal evolution of tumor cell populations. Science 194:23–28, 1976.
14. Rowley JD: Chromosome abnormalities in cancer. Cancer Genet and Cytogenet 2:175–198, 1980.
15. Rowley JD: Ph-positive leukemia, including chronic myelogenous leukemia. Clinics in Haematol 9:55–86, 1980.
16. Fialkow P, Denman A, Jacobson R, Leventhal M: Chronic leukemia: origin of some lymphocytes from leukemic stem cells. J Clin Invest 62:815–822, 1978.
17. Nowell P, Finan J, Glover D, Guerry D: Cytogenetic evidence for the clonal nature of Richter's syndrome. Blood 58:183–186, 1981.
18. Mark J: Rous sarcoma in mice: the chromosomal progression in primary tumors. Eur J Cancer 5:307–318, 1969.
19. Mitelman F: The chromosomes of fifty primary Rous rat sarcomas. Hereditas 69:155–162, 1971.
20. Boveri T: In: Zur Frage der Entstehung maligner Tumoren. Jenai Gustav Fischer Verlag, 1914.
21. Von Hansemann D: Über asymmetrische Zellteilung in Epithelkrebsen und deren biologische Bedeutung. Virchow Arch Pathol Anat Physiol 119:298–307, 1890.

22. Oksala T, Therman E: Mitotic abnormalities and cancer. In: Chromosomes and Cancer, German J (ed). New York: Wiley, 1974, pp 239–263.
23. Danes BS: Increased *in vitro* tetraploidy: tissue specific within the heritable colorectal cancer syndromes with polyposis coli. Cancer 41:2330–2334, 1978.
24. Otter M, Palmer C, Baehner R: Elevated sister chromatid exchange rate in childhood lymphoblastic leukemia. Proc Am Assoc Cancer Res 19:202, 1978.
25. Parshad R, Sanford KK, Tarone RE, Jones GM, Baeck AE: Increased susceptibility of mouse cells to fluorescent light-induced chromosome damage after long-term culture and malignant transformation. Cancer Res 39:929–933, 1979.
26. Shiraishi Y, Sandberg AA: Effects of various chemical agents on sister chromatid exchanges, chromosome aberrations, and DNA repair in normal and abnormal human lymphoid cells. J Natl Cancer Inst 62:27–33, 1979.
27. Sokova O, Volgareva G, Pogosiantz H: Effect of fluorafur on chromosomes of normal and malignant Djungarian hamster cells. Genetika 12:156–159, 1976.
28. Weiner F, Dalianis T, Klein G, Harris H: Cytogenetic studies on the mechanism of formation of isoantigenic variants in somatic cell hybrids. J Natl Cancer Inst 52:1779–1785, 1974.
29. German J: The association of chromosome instability, defective DNA repair, and cancer in some rare human genetic diseases. In: Human Genetics, Armendares S, Lisker R (eds). Amsterdam: Excerpta Medica, 1977, pp 64–68.
30. Hecht F, McCaw B: Chromosome instability syndromes. Prog Cancer Res Ther 3:105–123, 1977.
31. Setlow R: Repair deficient human disorders and cancer. Nature 271:713–717, 1978.
32. Li FP, Potter NU, Buchanan GR, Vawter G, Whang-Peng J, Rosen RB: A family with acute leukemia, hypoplastic anemia, and cerebellar ataxia: association with bone marrow C-monosomy. Am J Med 65:933–939, 1978.
33. Nowell P: Preleukemia: cytogenetic clues in some confusing disorders. Am J Pathol 89:459–476, 1977.
34. Seabright M: Patterns of induced aberrations in humans with abnormal autosomal complements. Chrom Today 5:293–297, 1976.
35. Law IP, Hollinshead AC, Whang-Peng J, Dean JH, Oldham RK, Herberman RB, Rhode MC: Familial occurrence of colon and uterine carcinoma and of lymphoproliferative malignancies. Cancer 39:1229–1236, 1977.
36. Miller OJ, Breg WR, Schmickel RD, Tretter W: A family with an XXXXY male, a leukemic male, and two 21 trisomic mongoloid females. Lancet ii:78–79, 1961.
37. Heston L: Alzheimer's disease, trisomy 21, and myeloproliferative disorders: associations suggesting a genetic diathesis. Science 196:322–323, 1977.
38. Loeb L, Battula N, Springgate C, Seal G: On mutagenic DNA polymerase and malignancy. In: Fundamental Aspects of Malignancy. Berlin: Springer, 1975, pp 243–246.
39. Hecht F, Kaiser McCaw B: Position effects in 8; 14 translocation in Burkitt's lymphoma. N Eng J Med 304:174–175, 1981.
40. McClintock B: The origin and behavior of mutable loci in maize. Proc Natl Acad Sci USA 36:344–355, 1950.
41. Sager R: Transposable elements and chromosomal rearrangements in cancer: a possible link. Nature 282:447–448, 1979.
42. Biedler JL, Spengler BA: Metaphase chromosome anomaly: association with drug resistance and cell-specific products. Science 191:185–187, 1976.
43. Balaban-Malenbaum G, Gilbert F: Double minute chromosomes and the homogeneously staining regions in chromosomes on a human neuroblastoma cell line. Science 198:739–742, 1978.

44. Passarge E, Bartram C: Somatic recombination as possible prelude to malignant transformation. In: Birth Defects: Original Article Series. New York: The National Foundation, 1976, pp 177–180.
45. Turleau C, Cabanis MO, De Grouchy J: Augmentation des échanges de chromatides dans les fibroblasts d'un enfant atteint de del(13)-rétinoblastome. Annales de Génétique 23:169–170, 1980.
46. Cairns J: The origin of human cancers. Nature 289:353–357, 1981.
47. Temin H: The DNA provirus hypothesis. Science 192:1075–1080, 1976.
48. Whang-Peng J, Knutsen T, Ziegler J, Leventhal B: Cytogenetic studies in acute lymphocytic leukemia: special emphasis in long-term survival. Med Pediatr Oncol 2:333–351, 1976.
49. Benedict W, Lange M, Greene J, Derencsenyi A, Alfi O: Correlation between prognosis and bone marrow chromosomal patterns in children with acute nonlymphocytic leukemia: similarities and differences compared to adults. Blood 54:818–823, 1979.
50. Hecht F, McCaw B: Chromosome instability syndromes. Prog Cancer Res Ther 3:105–123, 1977.
51. Levitt R, Pierre R, White W, Sickert R: Atypical lymphoid leukemia in ataxia-telangiectasia. Blood 52:1003–1011, 1978.
52. Saxon A, Stevens R, Golde D: Helper and suppressor T-lymphocyte leukemia in ataxia telangiectasia. N Eng J Med 300:700–704, 1979.
53. Nowell P, Shankey T, Finan J, Guerry D, Beas E: Proliferation, differentiation, and cytogenetics of chronic leukemic B lymphocytes cultured with motimycin-treated normal cells. Blood 57:444–451, 1981.
54. Prindull G, Jentsch E, Hansmann I: Fanconi's anaemia developing erythroleukemia. Scand J Haematol 23:59–63, 1979.
55. Berenblum I: Sequential aspects of chemical carcinogenesis in skin. In: Cancer: A Comprehensive Treatise, Becker FF (ed). New York: Plenum Press, 1975, pp 323–344.
56. Farber E, Cameron C: The sequential analysis of cancer development. Adv Cancer Res 31:125–225, 1980.
57. Orye E, Delbeke MJ: Clonal evolution in solid tumors in children. Oncol 29:520–533, 1974.
58. Balaban-Malenbaum G, Gilbert F: The proposed origin of double minutes from homogeneously staining region (HSR) marker chromosomes in human neuroblastoma hybrid cell lines. Cancer Gen and Cytogen 2:339–348, 1980.
59. Balaban-Malenbaum G, Gilbert F: unpublished.
60. Yunis JJ, Ramsay N: Retinoblastoma and subband deletion of chromosome 13. Am J Dis Child 132:161–163, 1978.
61. Balaban-Malenbaum G, Gilbert F, Nichols WW, Hill R, Shields J, Meadows AT: A deleted chromosome 13 in human retinoblastoma cells: relevance to tumorigenesis. Cancer Genet and Cytogenet (in press).
62. Balaban-Malenbaum G, Gilbert F, Nichols W: Abnormalities in chromosome 13 in direct preparations from human retinoblastoma. Am J Human Gen 32:62A, 1980.
63. Riccardi V, Sujansky E, Smith A, Francke U: Chromosomal imbalance in the aniridia-Wilms' tumor association: 11p interstitial deletion. Pediatrics 61:604–610, 1978.
64. Braun AC: The Cancer Problem. New York: Columbia University Press, 1969.
65. Di Berardino MA, King TJ: Transplantation of nuclei from the frog renal adenocarcinoma. II. Chromosomal and histologic analysis of tumor nuclear transplant embryos. Develop Biol 11:217–222, 1965.
66. Mintz B: Genetic mosaicism and *in vivo* analyses of neoplasia and differentiation. Ann Symp Cancer Res 30:27–53, 1978.
67. O'Hara M: Teratomas, neoplasia, and differentiation: a biological overview. I. The natural

history of teratomas. Invest Cell Pathol 1:39–63, 1978.

68. Kolber AR, Goldstein MN, Moore BW: Effect of nerve growth factor on the expression of colchicine-binding activity and 14-3-2 protein in an established line of human neuroblastoma. Proc Natl Acad Sci USA 71:4203–4207, 1974.

69. Mintz B, Illmensee K: Normal genetically mosaic mice produced from malignant teratocarcinoma cells. Proc Natl Acad Sci USA 72:3585–3589, 1975.

70. Meadows AT, Strong LC, Li SP, D'Angio DJ, Schweisguth O, Freeman AI, Jenkin RDT, Morris-Jones P, Nesbit ME: Bone sarcoma as a second malignant neoplasm in children: influence of radiation and genetic disposition. Cancer 46:603–606, 1980.

3. Cancer Cell Differentiation

DANIEL L. DEXTER and PAUL CALABRESI

Clinical and experimental oncologists have become increasingly aware that tumors can sometimes spontaneously differentiate to benign tissues and that cultured cancer cells can be triggered by chemical and biological inducers to undergo maturational events. These findings have encouraged investigations using maturational therapy in animal and human xenograft tumors. Moreover, studies to increase the efficacy of established modalities by preexposure of neoplastic cells, *in vitro* or *in vivo*, to differentiation-inducing agents would provide a logical extension of this approach. The prospect of clinical trials with biological modifiers, either alone or in combination with conventional treatment modalities, makes a concise review of cancer cell differentiation timely. In this chapter, investigations on the spontaneous, as well as on the experimentally-induced maturation of neoplastic cells are reviewed, and the clinical implications of cancer cell differentiation are discussed.

1 SPONTANEOUS DIFFERENTIATION OF TUMORS

1.1. Human Neuroblastoma

It has been known for some time that certain cancers can differentiate to more benign tissues. Spontaneous regressions of human neuroblastomas, with the conversion of neuroblastoma or ganglioneuroblastoma to benign ganglioneuroma, have been reported [1–4]. Dyke and Mulkey suggested that neoplastic cells had differentiated to benign ganglioneuroma cells, resulting in a control of the patient's disease [5]. Such examples from the clinical literature, although rare, have prompted investigators to consider whether triggering maturational events in cancers might lead to the arrest of proliferation, invasiveness or metastasis of human neoplasms [6, 7].

G. B. Humphrey et al. (eds.), Pancreatic Tumors in Children.
© *1982 Martinus Nijhoff Publishers, The Hague/Boston/London. ISBN-13:978-94-009-7617-7*

1.2. Murine Teratoma

Work with animal tumors has also provided evidence that tumors can spontaneously differentiate. Classical studies have been performed with the murine teratoma model, particularly in the laboratories of Stevens, and Pierce. Stevens has described the spontaneous differentiation of malignant teratocarcinomas to tissues containing thirteen distinct, normal tissue types. In some cases the neoplastic stem cells disappeared, leaving a benign cyst composed of a chaotic array of adult and fetal tissues [8, 9]. Kleinsmith and Pierce in an elegant study demonstrated that a single multipotential, neoplastic stem cell (embryonal carcinoma cell) from a mouse teratocarcinoma could give rise to the benign elements in the complex tumor commonly designated teratoma [10]. Work with this tumor, therefore, showed that neoplastic cells, in some instances, can differentiate into normal cells. More recently, Papaioannou et al., as well as Mintz and Illmensee have reported that the neoplastic stem cells of murine teratocarcinomas can participate in normal developmental processes when they are incorporated into blastocysts, which are then placed in pseudopregnant female mice. The offspring contain tissues that were derived from neoplastic, as well as from embryonic cells [11, 12]. These studies have provided compelling evidence that some tumor cells placed in an appropriate environment can mature to benign cells, which are able to participate in the normal processes of tissue and organ development.

2 INDUCTION OF DIFFERENTIATION IN CANCER CELLS

2.1. Biological Inducers

The mechanisms responsible for these changes in teratocarcinoma stem cells, or neuroblastoma cells, are unknown. Many investigators, however, have searched for factors or inducers that are produced by normal cells and might trigger maturational events in cancer cells. For many years, the laboratory of Sachs has been engaged in a study of a protein synthesized by normal cells that induces differentiation in leukemia cells. The protein, called macrophage granulocyte inducer (MGI), is synthesized and secreted by mouse fibroblasts and lung tissue [13, 14]. Medium conditioned by these cells and containing MGI, or the purified protein itself, can induce the differentiation of murine myelocytic leukemia cells to granulocytes and macrophages (for a review, see [7]). The search for naturally occurring molecules that can regulate and control cancer cell growth and differentiation represents an important effort, because identification of such substances would provide information on the aberrant regulation of cellular processes in neoplastic cells as well as on the mechanisms of biological induction of differentiation occurring in normal development.

2.2. Chemical Inducers

Although spontaneously regressing tumors have been reported, and biological inducers such as MGI have been isolated and studied, much of the effort towards causing the maturation of neoplastic cells has focused on the use of chemical inducers. These compounds are also sometimes referred to as maturational agents, or biological modifiers. The term biological inducer will be used in this chapter only to describe naturally occurring molecules synthesized by cells, such as the MGI protein. There have been, in the past ten years, numerous reports from many laboratories describing the differentiation–induction of many types of cancer cells with various chemical agents. The prototype for this approach has been the induction by dimethylsulfoxide (DMSO) of the erythroid program of differentiation in cultured Friend murine erythroleukemia cells (MEL cells). Initial work in the laboratory of Friend and co-workers [15, 16] has been extended by numerous investigators. Many differentiated features characteristic of erythrocytes rather than of leukemia cells have been reported in MEL cells following exposure to the polar solvent, DMSO. These include the appearance of hemoglobin, spectrin, globin mRNA, and an erythrocyte membrane antigen, in treated cells [15, 17–19]. Concomitant with this expression of differentiation markers, there is an alteration of the malignant phenotype of MEL cells exposed to DMSO. The treated cells are more benign as evidenced by loss of clonogenicity in soft agar, reduction in tumorgenicity, and the loss of proliferative capacity in culture [15, 20, 21]. DMSO-treated cells become post-mitotic, and thus can be described as terminally differentiated tumor cells.

Chemicals other than DMSO have been used to induce the differentiation of MEL cells. The list of inducing agents is long, and includes other polar solvents such as N,N-dimethylformamide (DMF) and N-methyl pyrolidinone, pyridine-N-oxide, various acetamides (notably hexamethylene bisacetamide), butyric acid or its sodium salt, ouabain, anticancer drugs such as thioguanine and actinomycin D, and prostaglandin E_1 [16, 22–28]. The fact that a large number of agents, many of which are structurally unrelated, induce MEL cell differentiation argues for the existence of more than one mechanism responsible for the maturation of these cells. Chemical inducers have been placed into categories or classes based on the ability or failure of any one agent to induce erythroid differentiation in MEL cells selected for their resistance to induction by another agent [29–31]. Moreover, results of studies in several laboratories, including our own, suggest that polar solvents such as DMSO and DMF induce the differentiation of MEL and other cancer cells by another mechanism than that involved with butyrate [24, 29, 31–34].

2.3. Neoplastic Cells Sensitive to Induction

While many workers have studied the effects of inducing-chemicals on MEL cells, other investigations have focused on different types of cultured cancer cells that are also inducible by these compounds. Again, an impressive list of many tumor cell types, which are sensitive to a variety of chemicals that modify the malignant phenotype, can be compiled. Mouse rhabdomyosarcoma, melanoma, fibrosarcoma, neuroblastoma, and teratoma cells [35–43], as well as hamster fibrosarcoma and melanoma cells [44, 45] have all been targets for inducing chemicals. Although these studies were performed with nonhuman tumor cells, there have been several reports on chemicals causing maturational events in human cancer cells. A human cancer cell line derived from a glioblastoma multiforme, which produces fibrosarcomas upon injection into nude mice, can be induced with hexamethylene bisacetamide to synthesize more adult type II collagen than is made by untreated cells [46]. DMSO has been shown to cause cilia formation in human lung cancer cells [47]. A number of compounds effect the maturation of cultured human promyelocytic leukemia cells to a phenotype more characteristic of macrophages [32, 48]. Different laboratories have reported the induction of differentiation in human melanoma cells by retinoic acid [49–51].

3 STUDIES ON HUMAN COLON CANCER CELLS

3.1. Alteration of Malignant Phenotype by DMF

Our laboratory has investigated the effects of inducing chemicals on cultured human colon cancer cells. The facts that colonic crypt cells divide every 24 hours and turn over every 3–4 days suggest that these cells may be targets in carcinogenesis occurring in the large bowel [52]. It has been postulated that colon cancers in man arise from transformed crypt cells, and therefore, colon carcinomas are stem cell tumors [53]. Such cells should in principle, be susceptible to maturational agents, and we have tested this hypothesis using four distinct human colon cancer cell lines and clones.

The following approach was used in our earlier studies. Alterations in the malignant phenotype of the cultured colon cancer cells after exposure to DMF were assessed, and changes in the levels of expression of certain marker molecules were also determined. DMF-treated colon cancer cells had increased doubling times, decreased saturation densities, a complete loss of colonogenicity in soft agar, and a markedly reduced tumorgenicity compared to their untreated counterparts [54]. Based on these criteria, the treated cells were more benign than untreated cells. DMF also caused significant changes in tissue- or organ-related markers in colon cancer cells [55]. Carcinoembryonic antigen expression was increased, and the H-gene-determined blood group cell surface product was decreased, after exposure to the polar solvent. Furthermore, the expression of the colonic mucoprotein antigens (CMAs) of Gold and Miller, isolated from normal (NCMA) and neoplastic (TCMA) colon tissues respectively [56, 57], was determined in these cell lines. DMF induced an increase in membrane-associated NCMA and a decrease in membrane-associated TCMA on cultured colon carcinoma cells. All the above effects are consistent with the induction by DMF of maturational changes in these cells [58]. Therefore, the polar solvent effects in human colon cancer cells an alteration of the malignant phenotype to a more benign phenotype with the occurrence of concomitant maturational events.

3.2. Combination of Inducing-Chemicals and Conventional Anticancer Modalities

More recently, we have begun to employ the following strategy for the use of inducing-chemicals in the experimental therapeutics of colon cancer [59]. Since differentiation-inducing chemicals cause changes in the antigenicity, enzyme activities, and hormone levels of cancer cells, such changes could potentially be utilized in approaches to the therapy of cancer. The exposure of neoplastic cells to inducers (biological modifiers), followed by conventional treatment modalities, could result in increased killing of neoplastic cells for the following reasons. Increased levels of antigens or hormone receptors might make tumor cells more responsive to hormones or immunotherapy, and a decrease in repair enzyme activities could sensitize cancer cells to ionizing radiation or hyperthermia. Increased activity of a drug-activating enzyme, or decreased activity of a drug-inactivating enzyme in cancer cells after exposure to an inducer could make the 'primed' tumor more responsive to the appropriate anticancer drug. In addition, membrane changes caused by polar solvent pretreatment of cancer cells [60] could result in a facilitated transport of a conventional antineoplastic agent into the cells.

Our findings that DMF induced an increase in expression of CEA and NCMA suggest that antigen targets can be modulated in human colon cancer cells. We have also demonstrated that DMF can induce the appearance of mouse mammary tumor virus (MMTV) antigen on mouse mammary tumor cells that had no detectable MMTV prior to DMF exposure [61]. Thus, there is evidence suggesting that prior exposure of cancer cells to biological modifiers may sensitize the cells to appropriate immuno-therapy.

Together with our colleagues, Dr. A.S. Glicksman and Dr. J.T. Leith, we have demonstrated that DMF can sensitize a relatively more radioresistant mouse mammary tumor cell subpopulation (clone 66) to X-irradiation [59]. The effect is observed primarily in the shoulder region of the survival curve, with D_q reduced from 2.8 Gy to 0.8 Gy. A relatively more radiosensitive subpopulation (clone 67), which we isolated from the same primary hetero-geneous mouse mammary tumor from which clone 66 was derived [62], was also pretreated with DMF, and the cells were X-irradiated. With this radio-sensitive line, there was no increased killing with exposure to the polar sol-vent. It is not known whether the increased responsiveness of clone 66 cells to X-rays after DMF pretreatment is due to a decreased ability of the cells to repair radiation damage, or to other causes. Studies currently underway at our Cancer Center suggest that DMF sensitizes human colon cancer cells to X-irradiation.

In collaboration with Dr. R.E. Parks, Jr. and Dr. G.W. Crabtree, we have initiated a study to determine whether DMF or sodium butyrate can modu-late the activities of purine metabolizing enzymes in cultured human colon cancer cells. Eleven enzymes were assayed in untreated cells and in cells treated with each agent [63]. The most striking result was obtained with DMF-treated clone A cells, derived from the heterogeneous human colon carcinoma line DLD-1 [54]. Adenosine deaminase (ADA) activity in clone A cells was reduced eleven-fold in DMF-treated compared to un-treated cells [34]. This suggests that colon cancer cells from some patients would be more responsive to adenosine analogs such as 8-azaadenosine or formycin, which are good substrates for ADA, after pretreatment with DMF. Our investigations therefore support the hypothesis that rational combinations of cytotoxic drugs, as well as irradiation, or immunomodula-tors, and biological modifiers might improve the efficacy of conventional antineoplastic therapy.

4. CLINICAL IMPLICATIONS OF CANCER CELL DIFFERENTIATION

In seeking the objective of using differentiation-inducing compounds to effect maturational therapy in a clinical setting, several mechanisms may be postulated. If the compound altered the phenotype of the cancer cells, inducing post-mitotic terminal differentiation, the disease might be con-trolled. Results with both chemical and biological inducers in laboratory models indicate that myelocytic leukemia in particular might be successfully treated this way [7, 32, 64, 65].

The major problem facing the clinical oncologist, however, remains the spectrum of solid tumors that accounts for the vast majority of deaths from neoplastic disease. Carcinomas of the breast, colon, pancreas, bladder, oropharynx, and lung, as well as melanoma, neuroblastoma, and brain tumors, should be considered as potential targets for maturational therapy. Carcinomas might be sensitive to maturational agents for several reasons. A marked reduction of proliferative rate may result from induction of a better differentiated phenotype. Significant growth-inhibiting effects, without concomitant toxicity, are commonly observed in cultures of cancer cells exposed to inducing-chemicals [35, 38, 44, 54]. The aggressive characteristics of tumor cells, i.e., their ability to invade and metastasize, may be attenuated by inducers. Compounds such as DMF, DMSO, and butyrate dramatically reduce or abolish the ability of cultured neoplastic cells to grow in soft agar, and also reduce the tumorigenicity of cancer cells [20, 35, 44, 54]. This loss of anchorage independence and reduction in tumorigenicity suggest that the other features of the transformed phenotype, including the invasive and metastatic capabilities of cancer cells, may be altered by the induction of the malignant phenotype to a more benign phenotype.

Maturational agents might also effect a conversion of distinct neoplastic subpopulations in a heterogeneous human solid tumor to a much more homogeneous population. We have suggested in a previous report that this could simplify therapy, since fewer agents would be needed because the tumor would not contain as many neoplastic subpopulations [66]. Our work with DMF and clones A and D isolated from the heterogeneous DLD-1 human colon cancer line supports this hypothesis. Although the clones differ significantly in several properties, such as clonogenicity in agar and expression of H-gene blood group substance, growth in DMF reduces or eliminates these differences [54, 55]. It is now well established that many human solid tumors are heterogeneous at the time of surgical resection [67–70], and heterogeneity has been identified as a major biological property responsible for frustrating antineoplastic therapy [66, 71, 72]. Should treatment with a biological modifier render a heterogeneous tumor more homogeneous, fewer modalities might be required to eliminate the better differentiated cancer cell population. This concept has played an important role in the development of our strategy that inducing-agents be used initially in the therapy of neoplastic disease, followed by treatment with conventional modalities [59]. Chemicals such as DMF, butyrate, or retinoic acid may be unable to convert all the cells present in a particular tumor to harmless, normal or benign phenotypes. If the altered phenotype of the modified cancer cell renders it more sensitive to antineoplastic drugs, ionizing radiation, heat, hormones, or immunotherapy, however, a greater cell kill will result than was obtained with the same dose of a conventional agent without pretreatment. Furthermore, elimination in a heterogeneous cancer of subpopulations with significant differential sensitivities to anticancer drugs or irradiation by a modifier-induced conversion to one phenotype could destroy a basic mechanism for developing drug resistance [66].

The use of biological modifiers in combination with conventional treatment modalities may be important for another reason. A number of studies with differentiation-inducing chemicals and cultured cancer cells have shown that the effects of some of these biological modifiers are reversible [33, 35, 36, 44, 54, 55, 73]. This implies that a patient undergoing maturational therapy would have to be maintained continuously on the inducing-chemical. This raises serious questions concerning the clinical usefulness of these biological modifiers as single agents. The use of biological modifiers to prime cancer cells for definitive treatment with drugs or ionizing radiation would eliminate this problem. The modifier would only have to be present long enough to sensitize the target neoplastic cell to the lethal conventional treatment. Moreover, even a limited exposure of an inducer that acts in a reversible fashion could have an effect on tumor growth. For example, an inhibition of the vascularization of the tumor during a brief exposure to an inducer might cause the tumor to become nutritionally compromised. We are currently studying the effect of DMF or butyrate on the growth of human colon tumor xenografts in nude mice, either as a single agent or in combination with antineoplastic drugs or X-irradiation, in order to test these concepts.

A number of human solid tumors appear to respond to biological modifiers. Among these, colon cancer may be a leading choice because we, and others [73], have already demonstrated that cultured human colon cancer cells are quite sensitive to phenotypic alterations by DMF, butyrate, or DMSO. Melanoma provides another reasonable candidate for this approach, because the disease is usually refractory to conventional therapy and because differentiation of human and mouse melanoma cells has been induced by a number of compounds [36, 37, 49–51].

Consideration of breast carcinoma raises the intriguing possibility that exposure of estrogen-receptor negative breast cancer cells to biological modifiers could convert these cells to an estrogen-receptor positive phenotype, making them better targets for hormonal therapy. Cancer of the urinary bladder and oropharynx represent other neoplasms that should be considered for studies with maturational agents. The multi-focal nature of these neoplasms provides increased difficulties for successful therapy. Topical administration of an inducer, such as DMF or DMSO, could provide a means for controlling progression of the disease, either alone or in combination with other modalities.

Certainly many of the theories presented in this chapter are still hypothetical, but accumulated experimental evidence suggests that biological modifiers may well play an increasingly important role in our design of innovative and effective treatment protocols. Furthermore, alterations in the malignant phenotype by chemical inducers will help us to better understand the biology of cancer cells, and to identify normal cells that are targets for carcinogens and promoters. Induction of differentiation in neoplastic cells elicits a salient concept in cancer biology: tumor tissues can be stimulated to undergo normal developmental and maturational events, and the induction of such events provides us with a potential means of controlling the disease.

ACKNOWLEDGEMENTS

The authors' investigations in this review were supported by USPHS grants CA23225, CA20892, and CA13943, from the National Cancer Institute.

REFERENCES

1. Cushing H, Wolbach SB: The transformation of a malignant paravertebral sympathicoblastoma into a benign ganglioneuroma. Am J Path 3:62–65, 1927.
2. Kissane JM, Ackerman LV: Maturation of tumors of the sympathetic nervous system. J Facul Radiol 7:109–114, 1955.
3. Fox F, Davidson J, Thomas LB: Maturation of sympathicoblastoma into ganglioneuroma. Cancer 12:108–116, 1959.
4. Visfeldt J: Transformation of sympathicoblastoma into ganglioneuroma. Acta Path Micro Scand 58:414–428, 1963.
5. Dyke PC, Mulkey DA: Maturation of ganglioneuroblastoma to ganglioneuroma. Cancer 20:1343–1349, 1967.
6. Pierce GB: The benign cells of malignant tumors. In: Developmental aspects of carcinogenesis and immunity, King TJ (ed). New York: Academic Press, 1974, pp 3–22.
7. Sachs L: The differentiation of myeloid leukemia cells: new possibilities for therapy. Br J Haematol 40:509–517, 1978.
8. Stevens LC: Experimental production of testicular teratomas in mice. Proc Natl Acad Sci USA 52:654–661, 1964.
9. Stevens LC: The biology of teratomas. Adv Morphog 6:1–31, 1967.
10. Kleinsmith LJ, Pierce GB: Multipotentiality of single embryonal carcinoma cells. Cancer Res 24:1544–1551, 1964.
11. Papaioannou VE, McBurney MW, Gordon RL, Evans MJ: Fate of teratocarcinoma cells injected into early mouse embryos. Nature 258:70–73, 1975.
12. Mintz B, Illmensee K: Normal genetically mosaic mice produced from malignant teratocarcinoma cells. Proc Natl Acad Sci USA 72:3585–3589, 1975.
13. Landau T, Sachs L: Characterization of the inducer required for the development of macrophage and granulocyte colonies. Proc Natl Acad Sci USA 68:2540–2544, 1971.
14. Burgess AW, Camakaris J, Metcalf D: Purification and properties of colony-stimulating factor from mouse lung-conditioned medium. J Biol Chem 252:1998–2003, 1977.

54

15. Friend C, Scher W, Holland JG, Sato T: Hemoglobin synthesis in murine virus-induced leukemic cells *in vitro*: stimulation of erythroid differentiation by dimethylsulfoxide. Proc Natl Acad Sci USA 68:378–382, 1971.

16. Scher W, Preisler HD, Friend C: Hemoglobin synthesis in murine virus-induced leukemic cells *in vitro*: III. Effects of 5-bromo-2'-deoxyuridine, dimethylformamide and dimethylsulfoxide. J Cell Physiol 81:63–70, 1973.

17. Eisen H, Bach R, Emery R: Induction of spectrin in erythroleukemic cells transformed by Friend virus. Proc Natl Acad Sci USA 74:3898–3902, 1977.

18. Preisler HD, Housman D, Scher W, Friend C: Effects of 5-bromo-2'-deoxyuridine on production of globin messenger RNA in dimethyl sulfoxide-stimulated Friend leukemia cells. Proc Natl Acad Sci USA 70:2956–2959, 1973.

19. Ikawa Y, Furusawa M, Sugano H: Erythrocyte membrane-specific antigens in Friend virus-induced leukemia cells. Bibl Haematol 39:955–967, 1973.

20. Preisler HD, Lutton JD, Giladi M, Goldstein K, Zanjani ED: Loss of clonogenicity in agar by differentiating erythroleukemic cells. Life Sci 16:1241–1252, 1975.

21. Gusella J, Geller R, Clarke B, Weeks V, Housman D: Commitment to erythroid differentiation by Friend erythroleukemia cells: a stochastic analysis. Cell 9:221–229, 1976.

22. Tanaka M, Levy J, Terada M, Breslow R, Rifkind RA, Marks PA: Induction of erythroid differentiation in murine virus infected erythroleukemia cells by highly polar compounds. Proc Natl Acad Sci USA 72:1003–1006, 1975.

23. Reuben RC, Wife RL, Breslow R, Rifkind RA, Marks PA: A new group of potent inducers of differentiation in murine erythroleukemia cells. Proc Natl Acad Sci USA 73:862–866, 1976.

24. Leder A, Leder P: Butyric acid, a potent inducer of erythroid differentiation in cultured erythroleukemic cells. Cell 5:319–322, 1975.

25. Bernstein A, Hunt DM, Crickley V, Mak TW: Induction by oubain of hemoglobin synthesis in cultured Friend erythroleukemic cells. Cell 9:375–381, 1976.

26. Gusella JF, Housman D: Induction of erythroid differentiation *in vitro* by purines and purine analogues. Cell 8:263–269, 1976.

27. Terada M, Epner E, Nudel V, Salmon J, Fibach E, Rifkind RA, Marks PA: Induction of murine erythroleukemia differentiation by actinomycin D. Proc Natl Acad Sci USA 75:2795–2799, 1978.

28. Tabuse Y, Furusawa M, Eisen H, Shibata K: Prostaglandin E_1, an inducer of differentiation of Friend erythroleukemia cells. Exp Cell Res 108:41–45, 1977.

29. Rovera G, Bonaiuto J: The phenotypes of variant clones of Friend mouse erythroleukemic cells resistant to dimethyl sulfoxide. Cancer Res 36:4057–4061, 1976.

30. Harrison PR, Rutherford T, Conkie D, Affara N, Sommerville J, Hissey P, Paul J: Analysis of erythroid differentiation in Friend cells using noninducible variants. Cell 14:61–70, 1978.

31. Rovera G, Surrey S: Use of hypersensitive variant clones of Friend cells in analysis of mode of action of inducers. Cancer Res 38:3737–3744, 1978.

32. Collins SJ, Ruscetti FW, Gallagher RE, Gallo RC: Terminal differentiation of human promyelocytic leukemia cells induced by dimethyl sulfoxide and other polar compounds. Proc Natl Acad Sci USA 75:2458–2462, 1978.

33. Dexter DL, Konieczny SF, Lawrence JB, Shaffer M, Mitchell P, Coleman JR: Induction by butyrate of differentiated properties in cloned murine rhabdomyosarcoma cells. Differentiation 18:115–122, 1981.

34. Dexter DL, Crabtree GW, Stoeckler JD, Savarese TM, Ghoda LY, Rogler-Brown TL, Parks RE Jr, Calabresi P: N,N-Dimethylformamide and sodium butyrate modulation of the activities of purine-metabolizing enzymes in cultured human colon carcinoma cells. Cancer Res

41:808–812, 1981.
35. Dexter DL: N,N-Dimethylformamide-induced morphological differentiation and reduction of tumorigenicity in cultured mouse rhabdomyosarcoma cells. Cancer Res 37:3136–3140, 1977.
36. Silagi S, Beju D, Wrathall J, De Harven E: Tumorigenicity, immunogenicity and virus production in mouse melanoma cells treated with 5-bromodeoxyuridine. Proc Natl Acad Sci USA 69:3443–3447, 1972.
37. Kreider JW, Wade DR, Rosenthal M, Densley T: Maturation and differentiation of B16 melanoma cells induced by theophylline treatment. J Natl Cancer Inst 54:1457–1467, 1975.
38. Borenfreund E, Steinglass M, Korngold G, Bendich A: Effect of dimethylsulfoxide and dimethylformamide on the growth and morphology of tumor cells. An NY Acad Sci 243:164–171, 1975.
39. Kimhi Y, Palfrey C, Spector I, Barak Y, Littauer UZ: Maturation of neuroblastoma cells in the presence of dimethylsulfoxide. Proc Natl Acad Sci USA 73:462–466, 1976.
40. Ishii DN, Fiback E, Yamasaki H, Weinstein BI: Tumor promoters inhibit morphological differentiation in cultured mouse neuroblastoma cells. Science 200:556–559, 1978.
41. Perreau PJ, Jacob H, Jacob F, Yaniv V: Tropomyosin synthesis accompanies formation of actin filaments in embryonal carcinoma cells induced to differentiate by hexamethylene bisacetamide. Proc Natl Acad Sci USA 76:1891–1895, 1979.
42. Strickland S, Mahdavi V: The induction of differentiation in teratocarcinoma stem cells by retinoic acid. Cell 15:393–403, 1978.
43. Jetten AM, Jetten MER: Possible role of retinoic acid binding protein in retinoid stimulation of embryonal carcinoma cell differentiation. Nature 278:180–182, 1979.
44. Leavitt J, Barrett JC, Crawford BD, Ts'o POP: Butyric acid suppression of the in vitro neoplastic state of Syrian hamster cells. Nature 271:262–265, 1978.
45. Avdalovic N, Aden D: Bromodeoxyuridine-(BrdUrd) and dimethylformamide-(DMF) induced changes in the surface of cultured hamster melanoma cells. Proc Am Assoc Cancer Res 19:195, 1978.
46. Rabson AS, Stern R, Tralka TS, Costa J, Wilczek J: Hexamethylene bisacetamide induces morphologic changes and increased synthesis of procollagen in cell line from glioblastoma multiforme. Proc Natl Acad Sci USA 74:5060–5064, 1977.
47. Tralka TS, Rabson AS: Cilia formation in cultures of human lung cancer cells treated with dimethyl sulfoxide. J Natl Cancer Inst 57:1383–1388, 1976.
48. Collins SJ, Bodner A, Tinge R, Gallo RC: Induction of morphological and functional differentiation of human promyelocytic leukemia cells (HL-60) by compounds which induce differentiation of murine leukemia cells. Int J Cancer 25:213–218, 1980.
49. Meyskens FL Jr, Fuller BB: Characterization of the effects of different retinoids on the growth and differentiation of a human melanoma cell line and selected subclones. Cancer Res 40:2194–2196, 1980.
50. Huberman E, Heckman C, Langenbach R: Stimulation of differentiated functions in human melanoma cells by tumor-promoting agents and dimethyl sulfoxide. Cancer Res 39:2618–2624, 1979.
51. Lotan R, Lotan D: Stimulation of melanogenesis in a human melanoma cell line by retinoids. Cancer Res 40:3345–3350, 1980.
52. Lipkin M, Bell B, Sherlock P: Cell proliferation kinetics in the gastrointestinal tract of man. I. Cell renewal in colon and rectum. J Clin Invest 42:767–776, 1963.
53. Pierce GB, Nakane PK, Hernandez-Martinez A, Ward JM: Ultrastructural comparison of differentiation of stem cells of murine adenocarcinomas of colon and breast with their normal counterparts. J Natl Cancer Inst 58:1329–1345, 1977.

54. Dexter DL, Barbosa JA, Calabresi P: N,N-Dimethylformamide-induced alteration of cell culture characteristics and loss of tumorigenicity in cultured human colon carcinoma cells. Cancer Res 39:1020-1025, 1979.
55. Hager JC, Gold DV, Barbosa JA, Fligiel Z, Miller F, Dexter DL: N,N-Dimethylformamide-induced modulation of organ- and tumor-associated markers in cultured human colon carcinoma cells. J Natl Cancer Inst 64:439–446, 1980.
56. Gold DV, Miller F: Characterization of human colonic mucoprotein antigen. Immunochemistry 11:369-375, 1974.
57. Gold DV, Miller F: Comparison of human colonic mucoprotein antigen from normal and neoplastic mucosa. Cancer Res 38:3204-3211, 1978.
58. Dexter DL, Hager JC: Maturation-induction of tumor cells using a human colon carcinoma model. Cancer 45:1178-1184, 1980.
59. Dexter DL, Leith JT, Crabtree GW, Parks RE Jr, Glicksman AS, Calabresi P: N,N-Dimethylformamide-induced modulation of responses of tumor cells to conventional anti-cancer treatment modalities. In: Maturation factors and cancer, Moore MAS (ed). New York: Raven Press (in press).
60. Lyman GH, Priesler HD, Papahadjopoulos D: Membrane action of DMSO and other chemical inducers of Friend leukemic cell differentiation. Nature 262:360-363, 1976.
61. Hager JC, Dexter DL, Calabresi P, Heppner GH: Heterogeneity of MMTV antigen expression and induction in mouse mammary tumor cells. Proc Am Assoc Cancer Res 20:61, 1979.
62. Dexter DL, Kowalski HL, Blazar BA, Fligiel Z, Vogel R, Heppner GH: Heterogeneity of tumor cells from a single mouse mammary tumor. Cancer Res 38:3174-3181, 1978.
63. Crabtree GW, Dexter DL, Stoeckler JD, Savarese TM, Ghoda LY, Rogler-Brown TL, Calabresi P, Parks RE Jr: Activities of purine metabolizing enzymes in human colon carcinoma cell lines and xenograft tumors. Biochem Pharmacol 30:793-788, 1981.
64. Honma Y, Kasukabe T, Okabe J, Hozumi M: Prolongation of survival times of mice inoculated with myeloid leukemia cells by inducers of normal differentiation. Cancer Res 39:3167-3171, 1979.
65. Sachs L: Control of normal cell differentiation and the phenotypic reversion of malignancy in myeloid leukemia. Nature 274:535-539, 1978.
66. Calabresi P, Dexter DL, Heppner GH: Clinical and pharmacological implications of cancer cell differentiation and heterogeneity. Biochem Pharmal 28:1933-1941, 1979.
67. Petersen SE, Bichel P, Lorentzen M: Flow cytometric demonstration of tumor cell subpopulations with different DNA content in human colorectal cancer. Eur J Cancer 15:383-386, 1978.
68. Siracky J: An approach to the problem of heterogeneity of human tumor-cell populations. Br J Cancer 39:570-577, 1979.
69. Hoshino T, Wilson CB: Cell kinetic analyses of human malignant brain tumors (gliomas). Cancer 44:956-962, 1979.
70. Vindelov LL, Hansen HH, Christensen IJ, Sprang-Thompson M, Hirsch FR, Hansen M, Nissen NI: Clonal heterogeneity of small-cell anaplastic carcinoma of the lung demonstrated by flow-cytometric DNA analysis. Cancer Res 40:4295-4300, 1980.
71. Heppner GH, Dexter DL, DeNucci T, Miller FR, Calabresi P: Heterogeneity in drug sensitivity among tumor cell subpopulations of a single mammary tumor. Cancer Res 38:3758-3763, 1978.
72. Dexter DL: Neoplastic subpopulations in carcinomas. Ann Clin Lab Sci 11:98-108, 1981.
73. Kim YS, Tsao D, Siddiqui B, Whitehead JS, Arnstein P, Bennett JJ, Hicks J: Effects of sodium butyrate and dimethylsulfoxide on biochemical properties of human colon cancer cells. Cancer 45:1185-1192, 1980.

4. Clinical Significance of Chromosome Abnormalities in Childhood and Adult Leukemia

YASUHIKO KANEKO and JANET D. ROWLEY

1. INTRODUCTION

Our knowledge of chromosome patterns in human leukemia has progressed remarkably since the advent of banding techniques, which permit the precise identification of each human chromosome and of parts of chromosomes as well. First, the nature of the Ph[1] chromosome in chronic myelogenous leukemia (CML) and the occurrence of nonrandom abnormalities in addition to the Ph[1] chromosome in the blastic phase of CML were established. Second, specific chromosome abnormalities in acute nonlymphocytic leukemia (ANLL) were identified; these changes were found to be closely related to certain clinical features and also to the morphology of the leukemic cells. More recently, nonrandom abnormalities in acute lymphoblastic leukemia (ALL) have been established, and their correlation with the clinical features of the disease has been clarified. We will review chromosome abnormalities that occur in leukemia, with emphasis on their clinical significance, and then we will delineate the similarities and the differences in the chromosome patterns observed in adult and childhood leukemia.

2. TECHNIQUES

Chromosomes of leukemic cells are usually obtained from bone marrow samples that are processed immediately or after 24-hour culture. If leukemic cells are present, peripheral blood can be processed by a short-term culture for 24 to 48 hours without mitogen. The chromosome pattern in the peripheral leukemic cells is identical to that in marrow cells, although the ratio of normal to abnormal cells may be different. Chromosomes are analyzed with regular Giemsa stain and with quinacrine-, Giemsa-, or reverse-banding techniques. We define abnormal clones as 2 or more metaphases with

G. B. Humphrey et al. (eds.), Pancreatic Tumors in Children.
© *1982 Martinus Nijhoff Publishers, The Hague/Boston/London.* ISBN-13:978-94-009-7617-7

identical extra chromosomes, 2 or more metaphases with identical structural rearrangements, or 3 or more metaphases with identical missing chromosomes.

The chormosomes are identified according to the International System for Human Cytogenetic Nomenclature (1978) [1], and the karyotypes are expressed as recommended under this system. The total chromosome number is indicated first, followed by the sex chromosomes, and then by the gains, losses, or rearrangements of the autosomes. A plus or minus sign before a number indicates a gain or a loss, respectively, of a whole chromosome, and after a number it indicates a gain or loss of part of a chromosome. The letters 'p' and 'q' refer to the short and long arms of the chromosome, respectively; 'i' stands for 'isochromosome'. Translocations are identified by 't', followed by the chromosomes involved in the first set of parentheses; the chromosome bands in which the breaks occurred are indicated in a second set. The morphology of the leukemic cells is designated according to the classification of the French-American-British (FAB) Cooperative Group [2].

3. CHROMOSOME PATTERNS IN ANLL DE NOVO

Our review includes 10 series of consecutive patients with ANLL *de novo* whose chromosomes were studied at diagnosis [3–12]. Of 402 patients, 199 (49.5%) had clonal chromosome abnormalities. We separated the patients into two age groups (less than 20 years old and 20 or more years old) and examined the percent of clonal abnormalities in each group. Of the 10 series, two which comprised a total of 115 patients [4, 5] were excluded

Table 1. Distribution of modal chromosome numbers in 141 ANLL patients 20 y.o. and older and that in 58 ANLL patients under 20 y.o.

	Modal chromosome number												
	42	43	44	45	46	47	48	49	50	51	52	53	54≦
Patients 20 y.o. and older [141]	2	5	8	37	41	33	7	2	0	2	0	0	4
Patients under 20 y.o. [58]			0	8[a]	25	14	5[b]	2	1[c]	1	1	1[c]	0

[a] One of the 8 patients had a t(13; 14) constitutional abnormality.
[b] Two of the 5 patients had Down's syndrome with an extra chromosome #21.
[c] Each patient had Down's syndrome with an extra chromosome #21.

from the evaluation because the age of the patients with a normal karyotype was not provided. Clonal abnormalities were found in 55 of 85 patients under 20 years old (y.o.) (64.7%) and in 102 of 202 patients 20 y.o. and older (50.5%). Thus, the incidence of abnormalities appears to be higher in the pediatric and adolescent patients than in adults. When we compare the distributions of modal chromosome numbers in the two groups of patients, we find that the incidence of hypodiploidy in the patients 20 y.o. and older is markedly higher than that in the patients less than 20 y.o. (Table 1). The reason for this difference will be discussed in Section 4.

Each of two translocations has been shown to be specifically associated with a particular type of ANLL. These are translocations that affect the long arms of chromosomes 8 and 21, t(8q−;21q+), and the long arms of chromosomes 15 and 17, t(15q+;17q−).

3.1. The 8;21 Translocation and Acute Myeloblastic Leukemia

The translocation involving the long arm of #8 and #21 is one of the common abnormalities in ANLL, which was observed in 23 of 199 aneuploid patients (11.6%) in this review. The incidence of this change appears to be almost equal in adults (15 of the 141 aneuploid patients: 10.6%) and in patients under 20 y.o. (8 of the 58 patients: 13.8%). The median age of patients with the t(8;21) is 26 years; this is much lower than the median age of patients with abnormalities other than the t(8;21), 50 years, or of those with a normal karyotype, 43 years [13]. The 8;21 translocation is frequently associated with loss of a sex chromosome (15 of the 23 patients in this review, and 16 of 48 patients reported at the Second International Workshop on Chromosomes in Leukemia (II IWC) [14]. A missing sex chromosome is otherwise relatively rare in ANLL.

The morphology of the leukemic cells in 43 patients with the t(8;21) was evaluated at the II IWC, and the cells were classified according to the FAB recommendations. The cells in all of the patients were identified as acute myeloblastic leukemia with maturation (M2). Other investigations have shown a high incidence of Auer rods in the myeloblasts (9 of the 15 patients of Kamada et al. [15] and all of the 32 patients of Trujillo et al. [16]). Other morphologic features of the granulocytes include maturation dysplasia, nucleoplasmic asynchrony, and abnormal lobation [15, 16]. The cells are positive for peroxidase [15, 16] and have a low alkaline phosphatase activity [15]. Another interesting aspect of this type of leukemia is that the patients appear to have a favorable prognosis; the complete remission rate and the survival were 74% and 11.5 months, respectively, at the II IWC [14] and 84.4% and 18.9 months, respectively, in the study by Trujillo et al. [16]. The prognostic as well as the diagnostic significance of the 8;21

translocation should be emphasized. Thus, although the presence of an abnormal karyotype is generally a sign of a poor prognosis, patients with this translocation do remarkably well.

3.2. The 15;17 Translocation and Acute Promyelocytic Leukemia

Another significant structural rearrangements is that observed in acute promyelocytic leukemia (APL). The FAB cooperative study group recently recognized that not all patients have the coarse granules which are usually found in APL (M3) and has added a category called the 'M3 variant' [17]. The most striking cytomorphologic features of this variant are the bilobed, multilobed, or reniform nuclear configuration and the relative scarcity of cells with heavy granulation or multiple Auer rods ('faggot' cells) [17]. The variant category was identified largely on the basis of the clinical features and of a specific chromosome abnormality, namely, the translocation involving the long arms of #15 and #17. The breakpoint in #15 appears to be distal to band q24, and that in #17 appears to be in q22 [18], but the exact breakpoints remain to be determined.

This translocation was observed in 8 of the 199 aneuploid patients (4%) in this review. Among 80 patients with APL evaluated at the II IWC [18], 33 had the t(15;17) (41%), 7 had other abnormalities, and the remaining 40 had a normal karyotype. Of the 33 patients with the t(15;17), 26 had typical APL, and 7 others had the variant form. This translocation has not been found in patients with other types of leukemia, or with other malignant diseases. The 15;17 translocation is, thus, a change that is specific for APL, although other karyotypic patterns can also be found in APL patients. The median survival of the 23 patients with t(15;17) was 1 month, that of the 10 with t(15;17) and additional abnormalities, 1.5 months, that of the 7 with other abnormalities, 5 months, and that of the 40 with a normal karyotype, 4 months [18]. This result suggests that the patients with t(15;17) have a poor prognosis compared with those who have other abnormalities or a normal karyotype. A recent clinical study of 31 APL patients whose karyotypes were not described, however, showed a median survival of 11 months [19], which was better than that of any group of APL patients evaluated at the II IWC [18]. More clinical information correlating karyotype and survival is required for evaluation of the prognostic significance of the t(15;17) in APL patients.

3.3. Other Abnormalities

An extra chromosome #8 was found in 28 of 141 aneuploid patients 20 y.o. and older (20%) and in 10 of the 58 aneuploid patients less than 20 y.o. (17%) among the 402 patients whom we reviewed. An extra chromosome #8 is the most frequent nonrandom abnormality and is seen in various

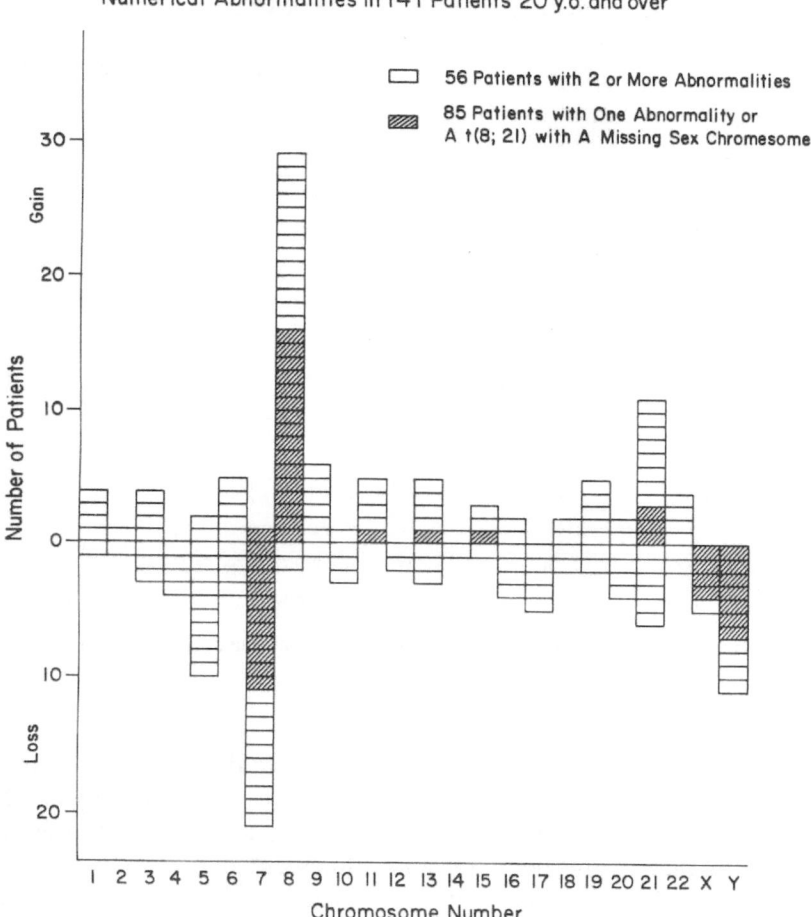

Numerical Abnormalities in 141 Patients 20 y.o. and over

☐ 56 Patients with 2 or More Abnormalities

▨ 85 Patients with One Abnormality or A t(8; 21) with A Missing Sex Chromosome

Figure 1. Histogram of numerical chromosome abnormalities at diagnosis in 141 patients 20 y.o. and older with acute nonlymphocytic leukemia (ANLL) *de novo.* The cross-hatched portion indicates the changes observed in the 85 patients who had one abnormality or a t(8;21) with a missing sex chromosome. 'One abnormality' indicates a rearrangement, such as +8 or t(15;17), without additional abnormalities.

hematologic malignancies, including ANLL, CML in blast phase [20], and even ALL [21]. A gain of #8 without other abnormalities, however, apparently occurs only in ANLL, including the preleukemic phase [22]. Thus, an isolated gain of #8 may be useful in distinguishing ANLL from ALL in patients whose leukemic cells are very immature and undifferentiated.

A loss of chromosome #7 with or without other abnormalities is also a common change in ANLL, including the preleukemic phase [27]. This

62

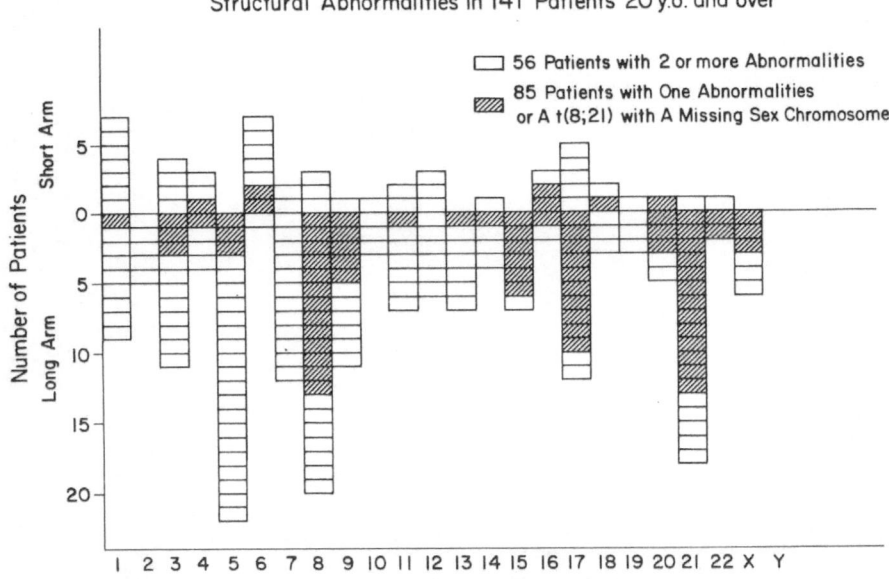

Figure 2. Histogram of structural chromosome abnormalities at diagnosis in 141 patients 20 y.o. and older with ANLL *de novo.*

abnormality was found in 23 of the 141 aneuploid patients 20 y.o. and older, and in only two of the 58 aneuploid patients less than 20 y.o. whom we reviewed. The incidence of this change in the adult patients was quite different from that in the pediatric and adolescent patients (Figures 1, 3). Borgström *et al.* [23] reported that the patients with monosomy 7 had a higher incidence of fever and infection and higher leukocyte counts at diagnosis than those who had ANLL and a normal karyotype in their leukemic cells. The high incidence of infection may indicate that chromosome #7 carries genes affecting neutrophil chemotactic function. Borgström *et al.* [23] also showed that these patients have a poor prognosis; the rate of complete remission was 12%, with a median survival of 5 months.

An abnormality of #11q was found in 7 patients [9–12] in this review, including one in our laboratory; all of these had a translocation involving #11 at band q22 or q23. The recipient chromosome was #19 in 4 of the patients, and #6, #9, and #13 each in one of them. With one exception, all patients had acute myelomonocytic leukemia (M4) or acute monocytic leukemia (M5); all were less than 20 y.o. and four of them were less than 2. Recently, Berger *et al.* [24] reported the chromosome patterns in 10 patients with acute monocytic leukemia (M5). Eight of the 10 patients had clonal

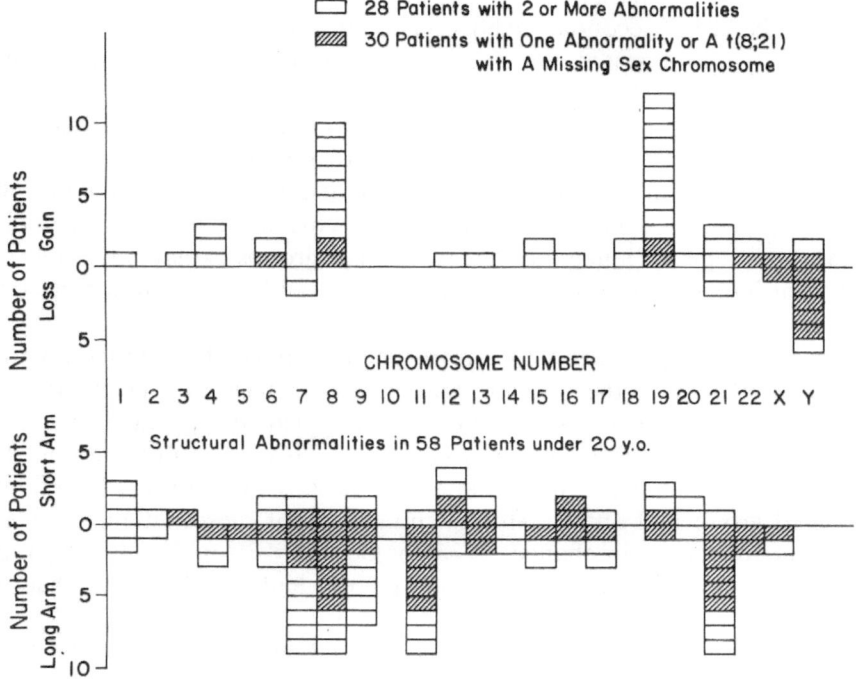

Figure 3. Histogram of numerical and structural chromosome abnormalities at diagnosis in 58 patients below 20 y. o. with ANLL *de novo.*

abnormalities, and five had rearrangements of the long arm of chromosome #11, but the rearrangements appeared to vary and to differ from those in our review. Thus, the 11q abnormality appears to be related to ANLL with monocytic differentiation, and the patients with this abnormality appear to be young.

4. CHROMOSOME ABNORMALITIES IN SECONDARY LEUKEMIA

An increased incidence of ANLL has been reported in patients who have had other malignant disorders that were treated with radiotherapy and/or chemotherapy. Rowley *et al.* reported on the cytogenetic patterns of bone marrow cells from 10 patients with secondary ANLL [25]. They recently combined these with an additional 17 patients who had a history of cytotoxic therapy for a previous malignant or nonmalignant disease [26]. Twenty-six of the 27 patients had an aneuploid clone of cells; 14 patients had a −5 or 5q−, and 18 patients had a −7. Rowley *et al.* concluded that a cytogenetic feature of secondary ANLL is an abnormal clone of cells, usually with a hypodiploid modal number, that is associated with the nonrandom loss of chromosome #5 and/or #7.

As shown in Figures 1–3, −5, 5q−, and −7 chromosome abnormalities are also seen in adult ANLL *de novo*, but are rare in childhood ANLL. These abnormalities are frequently found in patients who have smouldering acute leukemia [27] or erythroleukemia [11]. This difference in the incidence of these types of leukemia in different age groups explains the higher incidence of hypodiploidy in the patients 20 y.o. and older compared with that in the patients less than 20 y.o.

Mitelman *et al.* [6] reported on a retrospective study of 56 patients with ANLL *de novo*; 23 of the patients had histories suggesting occupational exposure to chemical solvents, insecticides, and petroleum products, whereas 33 had no history suggesting such exposure. Only 24.2% of the nonexposed group had clonal chromosomal abnormalities. In contrast, 82.6% of the exposed group had abnormalities, and 84.2% of these patients had at least one of four specific changes: −5 (or 5q−), −7 (or 7q−), +8, and +21. In the nonexposed group, only one patient had a −7 and one had a +21; none had −5 or +8.

The observation of a missing #5 or #7 in patients with secondary leukemia and in some patients with smouldering acute leukemia and erythroleukemia, the occurrence of these same aberrations in patients with ANLL *de novo* who may have had an exposure to mutagenic agents, and the absence of these abnormalities in childhood ANLL, all suggest the hypothesis that these particular chromosomes changes may identify acute leukemia associated with exposure to mutagenic agents.

Secondary leukemia is being reported with increasing frequency in children with ALL who were treated with cytotoxic agents and radiation [28–31]. A chromosome study of the leukemic cells of these children is especially important because, if they are found to have the chromosome patterns just described, such as hypodiploidy with −5, 5q−, and/or −7, which is rare in childhood ANLL *de novo*, this provides further support for the close association of particular karyotypes with cytotoxic agents. Of 4 children whose chromosomes were studied when they had secondary leukemia, one had 45,XX,−7 [29], another had 46,XX, t(3p−;11p+) [28], and two others had a normal karyotype [30]. Further study will resolve this important problem.

5. CHROMOSOME PATTERNS IN ALL

It has been reported that the most useful prognostic factors in childhood ALL are age, WBC count [32], and immunologic markers [33]. Age between 3 and 7 years, a WBC count less than $10,000/mm^3$ [32], and non-T, non-B markers [33] are good prognostic factors. Because of the difficulty of obtaining adequately banded chromosomes, reports describing the banding pattern have been fewer in ALL than in ANLL. Remarkable improvements, however, have been obtained in recent years. It is now possible to correlate the karyotype with other recognized prognostic factors and to show that data on chromosome patterns can increase the precision of previously recongized prognostic features.

This review includes data on the chromosome patterns of 30 ALL patients whom we have studied [34, 35], on patients described in recent reports [10, 21, 36–50], and on 330 patients evaluated at the Third International Workshop on Chromosomes in Leukemia (III IWC) [51]. Based on earlier studies, it appeared that chromosome abnormalities occurred in about one-half of the patients with ALL [21, 52], and hyperdiploidy was thought to be predominant among aneuploidies [21, 52]. The recent study of 330 ALL patients (adults, 173; children, 157) at the III IWC revealed that 65 % of the patients had clonal abnormalities. Of the 213 aneuploid patients, 34.8 % had pseudodiploidy, 24.5 %, hyperdiploidy, and 6.7 %, hypodiploidy. Our study on 30 ALL patients [35] also showed a high incidence of aneuploidy (66 %); pseudodiploidy was predominant (11 of the 20 aneuploid patients).

Although the karyotype in many of these patients may be very complex, certain patterns recur. It is now possible to analyze the clinical features of these patients, together with the morphology of the leukemic cells and the results of cell surface marker studies; this provides additional insight into the derivation of these malignant lymphoid cells.

5.1. 8;14 Translocation

A translocation involving the long arms of #8 and #14 has been detected in a large number of Burkitt tumors of both African and non-African origin, independent of whether they are EBV-positive or -negative [53, 54]. An apparently identical translocation has been observed in ALL patients with B-cell markers and in patients with L3-type leukemia cells [36–38], indicating that Burkitt lymphoma and most B-cell ALL of the L3-type are probably different manifestations of the same disease. Sixteen patients with this rearrangement were reported at the III IWC. There was an excess of males over females, and of adults over children. This group of patients had a high incidence of central nervous system involvement at diagnosis and a poorer prognosis (a median survival of 5 months) than any other group of patients classified according to chromosome patterns. With one exception, all patients in whom the immunologic markers of leukemic cells were identified had B-cell markers, and all but one had L3-type cells. In the exceptional patient, the leukemic cells had a pre-B-cell phenotype and were of the L1-type [39]; the morphology of the leukemic cells, however, changed to L3-type at relapse.

Recently, variant translocations have been reported in Burkitt lymphoma; these variants include a t(2;8)(p12-13;q24) [40] and a t(8;22)(q24;q11) [41]. Chromosome #8 was always involved in the translocation, with the breakpoint in band 8q23 or 24. This indicates that the common chromosome abnormality in Burkitt lymphoma is a rearrangement of #8q rather than that of #14q. The variant translocation t(2;8) was also found in an ALL patient with the L3-type [42].

The occurrence of variant translocations in Burkitt lymphoma may be analogous to that in CML; 92 percent of CML patients have a t(9;22), and the remaining 8 percent have variant translocation [55]. Chromosome #22, however, is involved in each translocation, with a break in band q11.

5.2. 14q+ Chromosome

A 14q+ chromosome is frequently observed in malignant lymphomas, particularly, although not exclusively, in those of B-cell origin [56]. Fifteen ALL patients at the III IWC [51] were reported to have a 14q+ chromosome that was not involved in a translocation with the terminal segment of chromosome #8. The excess of males over females and of adults over children is similar to that in the patients with t(8;14). One-half of the patients, however, had L2-type leukemic cells, and of the other half, one-fourth each had L1- and L3-type cells. The leukemic cells in about one-half of the patients had non-T, non-B immunologic markers, and the other one-half had B-cell markers. The 14q+ chromosome was due to a balanced translocation in 6 patients, in 4 of whom the donor chromosome was identified as #11. The t(11;14) is one of the common abnormalities seen in malignant lymphoma, poorly differentiated lymphocytic type [56], suggesting that there is a relationship between it and ALL with a 14q+ chromosome. The latter group of patients also had a poor prognosis; the complete remission rate was 53%, with a median survival of 9 months [51].

5.3. 4;11 Translocation

A translocation involving the long arms of #4 and #11 was observed in 4 of 52 ALL patients of Van den Berghe et al. [43], 4 of 34 patients of Prigogina et al. [10], and one of 31 patients of Oshimura et al. [21], but in none of our 30 ALL patients [35]. According to the report on 18 patients with this change who were evaluated at the III IWC [51], these patients had very high leukocyte counts (median WBC, 183,000/mm^3). The leukemic cells were L1-type in 7 patients, L2-type in 7, and L3-type in one patient. Of 8 patients in whom immunologic markers were tested, 7 had non-T, non-B ALL, and one had T-cell ALL. These patients had a very poor prognosis; the complete remission rate was 67%, and the median survival was 7 months. One-half of the patients were adults; the other one-half were children most of whom were less than 1 year old. The association of the 4;11 translocation with neonatal or early-childhood ALL is particularly interesting in view of the low incidence of ALL in this age group.

5.4. Near-Haploid ALL

The occurrence, in ALL, of leukemic cells with a near-haploid number of chromosomes is rare. Five such cases have been published [44–48], and two new cases were presented at the III IWC [51]. There were 4 males and 3 females; five were children or adolescents, and 2 were adults. These 7 patients had a remarkably consistent chromosome pattern. The chromosome number of the near-haploid clone ranged from 26 to 36 (median, 28). A boy reported by Prieto et al. [46] is presumed to have had the karyotype 26,XY,+41,+21, although the chromosomes were not banded. In addition to a haploid set, +21 was seen in all patients, +10 and +18 in 6, +X or +Y in 5, +6 in 4, +1, +19, and +22 in 3, and +14 in 3. Patients in four [44, 45, 47, 48] of the five published reports had a variable percentage of cells that contained double the number of chromosomes of the near-haploid line. Of the 2 patients for whom immunologic markers were tested, both had non-T, non-B ALL [45, 48]; one was identified as having common ALL [45]. Two patients had no response to chemotherapy [46, 47], whereas three others achieved a complete remission [44, 45, 48]; however, all three had a relapse after 6 to 16 months of remission. The median survival was 9 months. Thus, ALL with near-haploidy may be a unique subgroup of ALL, with a prognosis that is poor compared with that for other types of non-T, non-B ALL.

A near-haploid clone has also been found in 4 patients in the blast phase of CML [57–60]. In addition to a haploid set, three of the 4 patients had +21, another three had +X or +Y, and two had +14 and +18. All retained the Ph^1 chromosome. Thus, these karyotypes showed some similarities to those of ALL patients with near-haploidy, although they seemed to be more variable. Two of the patients appeared to have a lymphoblastic crisis; therefore, the karyotype may reflect the lymphoid character of the blast cells.

5.5. Hyperdiploidy with 50 to 60 Chromosomes

The karyotype of some patients is characterized by many extra chromosomes and few structural abnormalities. Chromosome numbers usually range from 50 to 60, and a few patients may have up to 65 chromosomes. Although identical karyotypes are rarely found, certain additional chromosomes are commonly seen. Among 30 patients, including 22 children and 8 adults evaluated at the III IWC [51], +21 was seen in 22, +6 in 15, +18 in 14, +14 in 11, +4 in 10, and +10 in 10 patients. If we compare the additional chromosomes that were common in this group with additional chromosomes in the 7 patients reviewed in Section 5.5 who had the haploid complement, the similarities are remarkable, since the most consistent changes in the latter group are +10, +18, and +21.

The median age of the 22 children with this abnormality was 3 years, and that of all 30 patients was 5 years, which was less than that of patients with other abnormalities. The WBC count in patients with hyperdiploidy was low, with a median of 6,000/mm^3; it was below 10,000/mm^3 in more than half of the patients. The L1- and L2-types were seen in about equal numbers, and all patients had non-T, non-B ALL. A good prognosis for this group was reported by Secker Walker et al. [49] and Kaneko et al. [50]. We found hyperdiploidy with 50 to 60 chromosomes in 3 of the 30 ALL patients; all continue to be in their first remission (46 days to 1095 days) [35]. The complete remission rate and the median survival of the 30 patients evaluated at the III IWC [51] were 87% and 34 months, respectively. Thus, in patients who have hyperdiploidy with more than 49 chromosomes, all of the previously recognized factors, including age between 3 and 7 years, low WBC count, and non-T, non-B markers, are present that indicate a good prognosis. It should be emphasized that the median survival of the hyperdiploid patients, including both children and adults, is longer than that of patients with a normal karyotype.

5.6. Ph^1 Chromosome in ALL

A Ph^1 chromosome, which is formed by a reciprocal translocation between #22 and #9 or various other chromosomes, is seen in patients with ALL, as well as in patients with CML (see next section). Of the 39 patients evaluated at the III IWC [51], thirty were adults and nine were children. The incidence of Ph^1-positive patients with ALL was 5.7% for children and 17.3% for adults; the incidence previously reported was 2.0% for children [61] and 25% for adults [62]. Thus, the Ph^1 chromosome is the most frequent rearrangement in adult ALL. Thirty-six patients had the typical t(9q+ ; 22q−), and the remaining 3 had variant translocations; the incidence of the variant form was 8%, which is similar to that observed in CML patients [55]. About one-half of the patients showed abnormalities in addition to the Ph[1] chromosome. These additional changes were quite variable, and the usual changes seen in the blast crisis of CML were absent except for +8 in one case. The patients had a high leukocyte count (median WBC, 34,000/mm^3), and all had non-T, non-B ALL. The complete remission rate was 55%. The median survival was 9 months, reflecting the poor prognosis for these patients. By identifying this chromosome abnormality, one can detect individuals in the non-T, non-B category who have a poor prognosis.

6 CHROMOSOME PATTERNS IN CML

6.1. The Ph[1] Chromosome in CML

Among all hematologic malignancies, chronic myelogenous leukemia (CML) has been studied most extensively with regard to chromosome abnormalities [20]. Of all Ph[1]-positive CML patients, 92 percent had a Ph[1] chromosome due to the t(9q+; 22q−), and the remaining 8 percent had a Ph[1] resulting from unusual rearrangements [55]. Chromosome abnormalities in addition to the Ph[1] translocation are found in up to 22 percent of CML patients in the chronic phase [55]. These abnormalities include an extra #8, i(17q), a second Ph[1], and loss of the Y chromosome [55]. When patients enter the blast phase, about 20 percent appear to retain the 46, Ph[1] cell line unchanged, whereas the other 80 percent show additional changes [55]. The pattern of additional abnormalities is similar to that found in CML patients in the chronic phase. An additional change detected at the time of diagnosis of the chronic phase does not seem to carry a substantially poorer prognosis than the typical 46,Ph[1] pattern [63]. A change in karyotype, however, is generally considered to be a grave prognostic sign [63].

Because of the low percentage of CML among childhood leukemias (2 to 5%), banded karyotypes have been reported for only 15 children with Ph[1]-positive CML, including 5 patients from our laboratory [61, 64–66]. Their ages ranged from 3 to 14 years; 8 were male and 7 female. Eleven of the 15 patients had the usual translocation, t(9q+; 22q−), and four had variant forms. There appears to be no difference in the clinical and hematologic features between adults and children who have Ph[1]-positive CML.

A lymphoid blast crisis has been reported in some Ph[1]-positive CML patients [67]. Moreover, some patients who had what appeared to be ALL at the onset subsequently developed typical features of CML when they entered remission after chemotherapy [68]. The morphologic, cytochemical, and immunologic features of the lymphoblasts in these patients are quite similar to those in Ph[1]-positive ALL. There are, however, some differences in the chromosome findings between Ph^1-positive ALL and CML in lymphoid blast crisis [20, 69]. The former patients usually have normal cells as well as Ph^1-positive cells in the marrow at diagnosis, and the Ph^1-positive cells disappear when these patients achieve a complete remission. On the other hand, the latter patients usually have only Ph^1-positive cells in the marrow at the time of blast crisis; if additional abnormalities are superimposed in blast cells, these disappear if the patient enters remission, but the original Ph^1 cell line remains. Recently, Catovsky [70] suggested that, when a Ph^1-positive 'lymphoid' clone has been eliminated by therapy, it may be followed by a Ph^1-positive (leukemic) or a Ph^1-negative (normal) stem cell that moves into the stem cell compartment where hemopoietic differentiation and maturation occur. Which of these stem cells succeeds the Ph^1-positive 'lymphoid' clone depends on the number of generations of stem cells that are affected by the Ph^1 aberration. The question whether Ph^1-positive acute leukemia and CML are different diseases is unresolved, but there is good reason to view them as different manifestations of the same malignant process.

6.2. 'Juvenile-type' CML

In comparison to Ph^1-positive CML, which is well-defined entity 'juvenile' CML seems to have less specific characteristics. Smith and Johnson [71] described the most valuable parameters for distinguishing 'juvenile' CML from 'adult' (Ph^1-positive) CML; these include the WBC count, the presence of thrombocytopenia or thrombocytosis, and the bone marrow myeloid–erythroid (M:E) ratio. Patients with 'juvenile' CML had moderately increased WBC counts (median, $29,500/mm^3$), thrombocytopenia, and a normal M:E ratio whereas those with Ph^1-positive CML had greatly increased WBC counts (median, $250,000/mm^3$), thrombocytosis, and a high M:E ratio. On the other hand, Altman et al. [72] proposed that 'juvenile' CML should be classified as a variant of myelomonocytic leukemia. There have been only 5 reported patients with 'juvenile' CML whose karyotypes were analyzed with banding [65, 72–74]. Their ages ranged from 16 months to 5 years. Four were male and one female. Only one of the patients had a normal karyotype [72]. Of the 4 patients with an abnormal karyotype, three had reciprocal translocations, namely, $t(3q+;7q-)$ [72], $t(3p-;11p+)$ [73], or $t(2q-;8q+)$ [74], and the fourth had a $45,X,-Y$ karyotype [65]. It is difficult to reach any conclusion on the chromosome pattern at this point. The karyotype in 'juvenile' CML seems to be quite variable, the only consistent finding being the absence of a Ph^1 chromosome.

7. DOWN'S SYNDROME AND ACUTE LEUKEMIA

It is generally accepted that children with Down's syndrome (DS) are at increased risk of acute leukemia (AL) compared with those without DS [75]. Some DS neonates have hepatomegaly, splenomegaly, and leukocytosis with a substantial percentage of myeloblasts; these features are indistinguishable from those of acute leukemia, but disappear within a few months without treatment [76, 77]. Some consider these features to be those of acute leukemia [76]; others, however, regard them as a 'transient leukemoid reaction' [77]. Recently, Brodeur et al. [78] reported on a phenotypically normal 3-day old boy with the above symptoms. A chromosome study revealed trisomy 21 in all blood and bone marrow cells. However, only 4% of cultured skin fibroblasts were trisomic and the other 96% were normal, indicating mosaicism. At the age of 100 days when the clinical and hematologic features returned to normal, all of the cells in the bone marrow and the majority of the cells (76%) in the blood had a normal karyotype. This case suggests that the cells with an extra chromosome #21 may temporarily gain a proliferative advantage over the normal cells and thus could cause the transient leukemoid reaction seen in some DS newborns.

We recently studied 3 DS patients with ANLL and reviewed the data on 40 other published cases in which chromosomes in leukemic cells were studied [79]. Banding was used to identify abnormalities in only 7 of these patients, including 3 of ours. Sixteen of these 43 patients had the karyotype 47,XX,+21 or 47,XY,+21, and the remaining 27 had chromosome abnormalities in addition to the expected trisomy 21. Thus, chromosome abnormalities were found in 63% of DS patients with AL; this is similar to the incidence in other patients with AL. The distribution of the modal chromosome number in 19 DS ANLL patients with an abnormal karyotype and that in 38 non-DS ANLL children with an abnormal karyotype reported in the literature were compared. The distribution pattern differed considerably in the two groups. Whereas hypodiploidy or pseudodiploidy was seen in one-half of the non-DS patients, neither was present in the DS patients. One-half of the DS patients had 2 or more extra chromosomes; this finding was relatively rare in non-DS children with ANLL. We also compared the pattern of extra chromosomes in the 2 groups. The incidence of extra C, F, and G chromosomes in the DS group was markedly higher than that in the non-DS group. Although karyotypes were examined with banding in only 5 of the 19 DS children, the result suggests that +C, +F, and +G may be +8, +19, and +21 and +22. One of our patients with the karyotype 50,XX,+6,+19,+21,+22 had leukemic blasts in an early stage of myeloid differentiation. Similar morphologic features were reported in 3 other DS patients who had a related karyotype which was characterized by hyperdiploidy with 3 or more extra chromosomes; these included a #19 and a #22, or an F and a G. Our other 2 patients whose cells were examined with banding had an extra chromosome #8, and they had several cytologic and clinical features in common. Their leukemic blasts were also arrested in early myeloid differentiation. One of 3 DS ANLL patients with +C in our review had similar primitive cells. Our study showed that almost all chromosome abnormalities in DS with ANLL involve hyperdiploidy. Abnormalities of +8 and of +19, +22 may be associated with AL in an early stage of myeloid differentiation.

The high incidence of AL in DS and the apparent temporary proliferative advantage of +21 cells in some DS neonates, together with the frequent occurrence of +21 in the leukemic cells of non-DS patients with ALL or ANLL, suggest that chromosome 21 carries genes related to hematopoiesis or leukemogenesis. Future gene mapping studies as well as clinical observations may clarify the exact role of an extra #21 chromosome in this process.

8. PROGNOSTIC IMPLICATION OF CHROMOSOME ABNORMALITIES IN ACUTE LEUKEMIA

A correlation of karyotypes with survival of patients with ANLL was first reported by Sakurai and Sandberg [80]. They observed that patients, primarily adults, who had only abnormal metaphases in the bone marrow (AA patients) had very short survival times as compared with those of patients who had both abnormal and normal (AN patients) or only normal metaphases (NN patients). This observation was confirmed with banding studies in adults by Nilsson et al. [81], Golomb et al. [82], and the First International Workshop on Chromosomes in Leukemia [83], and in children by Benedict et al. [8]. Although these studies provided significant information, some problems still remain. First, the number of cells analyzed with banding is usually less than 15 per patient because of technical difficulties, such as an inadequate number of cells and lack of time. If we increase the number of banded cells that are analyzed, we may find normal metaphases in a bone marrow in which only abnormal cells had been found, and therefore AA patients may have to be reclassified as AN patients. In fact, when one of us analyzed more than 50 banded cells from each patient, normal metaphases were found in the bone marrow of 2 patients whom all 15 cells initially studied had been abnormal. On the other hand, recent studies have demonstrated that some patients whose directly processed marrow aspirates showed only normal metaphases had abnormal metaphases in marrow aspirates cultured for 24 to 48 hours [84]. Thus, some NN patients may be reclassified as AN patients when better techniques for detection of abnormal metaphases are used. Moreover, the use of elongated chromosomes will help to reveal subtle deletions or translocations that are overlooked at present. The findings depend on whether or not the patients received optimal chemotherapy. Since current chemotherapy of ANLL patients is very aggressive, their survival may be greatly influenced by the supportive care available and by the skill of the therapist. When these questions are resolved, the prognostic implications of the frequency of abnormal mitotic cells will become more accurate.

Among ANLL patients with an abnormal karyotype, those with an 8;21 translocation have a high remission rate and a long survival [14, 16]. The hypodiploid patients with -5, 5q$-$, and/or -7 appear to have a low remission rate and a short survival [23, 27].

Among adult ALL patients, NN patients had longer survival than did AN or AA patients [51]. There was, however, no difference between the survival of AN patients and that of AA patients [51]. Among childhood ALL patients, there was no difference of survival times in NN, AN, and AA patients [51]. All consistent abnormalities, including a Ph[1] chromosome, t(8;14), a 14q$+$ chromosome, t(4;11), and near-haploidy, appear to be associated with a poor prognosis [51]. Hyperdiploidy with 50 and more chromosomes is an exception, since it is associated with a good prognosis [51].

9. DIFFERENCES IN KARYOTYPE IN CHILDREN AND IN ADULTS

There seem to be no consistent chromosome abnormalities which are specific for childhood leukemia or adult leukemia. Some abnormalities may be prevalent in a given age group of patients. The 8;21 and 15;17 translocations in ANLL occur both in children and in adults; however, these are uncommon in patients more than 50 years old. In contrast, hypodiploidy with -5, 5q$-$, and/or -7 is rare in children, but is frequent in adults over age 50. Among the karyotypes in ALL, t(9;22), t(8;14), and t(4;11) are seen both in children and in adults. Hyperdiploidy with 50 or more chromosomes and near-haploidy are more common in children than in adults. These differences in karyotype in children and in adults may reflect different etiologic factors in each type of leukemia.

10. CONCLUSION

We have reviewed the evidence which shows that the karyotype in human leukemia is closely correlated with clinical and hematologic features. A chromosome study is now essential for the diagnosis and prediciton of the prognosis in leukemia patients. We also showed that some chromosome abnormalities were prevalent in certain age groups. In the future, when we have a more complete human gene map, we will understand the basis of these correlations and the etiologic significance of the chromosome changes that we have observed.

ACKNOWLEDGMENTS

The authors thank Elisabeth Lanzl for editorial review, and Fay Yates for secretarial assistance.

This work was supported in part by a contract from the U.S. Department of Energy, No. DE-AC02-80EV10360, by Grants CA-16910 and CA-19266 from the National Cancer Institute, Department of Health and Human Services, and by The University of Chicago Cancer Research Foundation.

REFERENCES

1. An International System for Human Cytogenetic Nomenclature (1978): Cytogenet Cell Genet 21:309–404, 1978.
2. Bennett JM, Catovsky D, Daniel MT, Flandrin G, Galton DAG, Gralnick NR, Sultan C: [French-American-British (FAB) Cooperative Group] Proposals for the classification of the acute leukaemias. Br J Haematol 33:451–458, 1976.
3. Rowley JD, Potter D: Chromosomal banding patterns in acute nonlymphocytic leukemia. Blood 47:705–721, 1976.
4. Oshimura M, Hayata I, Kakati S, Sandberg AA: Chromosomes and causation of human cancer and leukemia. XVII. Banding studies in acute myeloblastic leukemia (AML). Cancer 38:748–761, 1976.
5. Philip P, Jensen MK, Killmann SA, Drivsholm A, Hansen NE: Chromosomal banding patterns in 88 cases of acute nonlymphocytic leukemia. Leukemia Res 2:201–212, 1978.
6. Mitelman F, Brandt L, Nilsson PG: Relation among occupational exposure to potential mutagenic/carcinogenic agents, clinical findings, and bone marrow chromosomes in acute nonlymphocytic leukemia. Blood 52:1229–1237, 1978.
7. Rowley JD: The cytogenetics of acute leukaemia. Clin Haematol 7:385–406, 1978.
8. Benedict WF, Lange M, Greene J, Derenscenyi A, Alfi OS: Correlation between prognosis and bone marrow chromosomal patterns in children with acute nonlymphocytic leukemia: Similarities and differences compared to adults. Blood 54:818–823, 1979.
9. Morse H, Hays T, Rose B, Robinson A: Acute nonlymphoblastic leukemia in childhood: High incidence of clonal abnormalities and nonrandom changes. Cancer 44:164–170, 1979.
10. Prigogina EL, Fleischman EW, Puchkova GP, Kulagina OE, Majakova SA, Balakirev SA, Frenkel MA, Khvatova NV, Peterson IS: Chromosomes in acute leukemia. Hum Genet 53:5–16, 1979.
11. Hagemeijer A, Kahlen K, Abels J: Cytogenetic follow-up of patients with non-lymphocytic leukemia. II. Acute non-lymphocytic leukemia. Cancer Genet Cytogenet 3:109–124, 1981.

12. Kaneko Y, Rowley JD, Variakojis D, Maurer HS, Moohr JW: Chromosomes in childhood acute nonlymphocytic leukemia (in press).
13. Rowley JD: Association of specific chromosome abnormalities with type of acute leukemia and with patient age. Cancer Res. 41:3407-3410, 1981.
14. Second International Workshop on Chromosomes in Leukemia (1979): Cytogenetic, morphologic, and clinical correlations in acute nonlymphocytic leukemia with t(8q−; 21q+). Cancer Genet Cytogenet 2:99-102, 1980.
15. Kamada N, Okada K, Oguma N, Tanaka R, Mikami M, Uchino H: C-G translocation in acute myelocytic leukemia with low neutrophil alkaline phosphatase activity. Cancer 37:2380-2387, 1976.
16. Trujillo JM, Cork A, Ahearn MJ, Youness EL, McCredie KB: Hematologic and cytologic characterization of 8/21 translocation acute granulocytic leukemia. Blood 53:695-706, 1979.
17. Bennett JM, Catovsky D, Daniel MT, Flandrin G, Galton DAG, Gralnick HR, Sultan C: A variant form of hypergranular promyelocytic leukaemia (M3). Br J Haematol 44:169-170, 1980.
18. Second International Workshop on Chromosomes in Leukemia (1979): Chromosomes in acute promyelocytic leukemia. Cancer Genet Cytogenet 2:103-107, 1980.
19. Mertelsmann R, Thaler HT, To L, Gee TS, McKenzie S, Schauer P, Friedman A, Arlin Z, Cirrincione C, Clarkson B: Morphological classification, response to therapy, and survival in 263 adult patients with acute nonlymphoblastic leukemia. Blood 56:773-781, 1980.
20. Rowley JD: Ph¹-positive leukemia, including chronic myelogenous leukemia. *Clinics in Haematol* 9: 55-86, 1980.
21. Oshimura M, Freeman AI, Sandberg AA: Chromosomes and causation of human cancer and leukemia. XXVI. Banding studies in acute lymphoblastic leukemia (ALL). *Cancer* 40: 1161-1172, 1977.
22. Second International Workshop on Chromosomes in Leukemia (1979). Chromosomes in preleukemia. Cancer Genet Cytogenet 2:108-113, 1980.
23. Borgström GH, Teerenhovi L, Vuopio P, de la Chapelle A, Van Den Berghe H, Brandt L, Golomb HM, Louwagie A, Mitelman F, Rowley JD, Sandberg AA: Clinical implications of monosomy 7 in acute nonlymphocytic leukemia. Cancer Genet Cytogenet 2:115-126, 1980.
24. Berger R, Bernheim A, Weh H-J, Daniel M-T, Flandrin G: Cytogenetic studies on acute monocytic leukemia. Leukemia Research 4:119-127, 1980.
25. Rowley JD, Golomb HM, Vardiman J: Nonrandom chromosomal abnormalities in acute nonlymphocytic leukemia in patients treated for Hodgkin's disease and non-Hodgkin's lymphomas. Blood 50:759-770, 1977.
26. Rowley JD, Golomb HM, Vardiman JW: Nonrandom chromosome abnormalities in acute leukemia and dysmyelopoietic syndrome in patients with previously treated malignant disease. Blood 58:759-767, 1981.
27. Streuli RA, Testa JR, Vardiman JW, Mintz U, Golomb HM, Rowley JD: Dysmyelopoietic syndrome: Sequential clinical and cytogentic studies. Blood 55:636-644, 1980.
28. Ravindranath Y, Inoue S, Considine B, Lusher J, Zuelzer WW: New leukemia in the course of the therapy of acute lymphoblastic leukemia. Am J Hematol 5:211-223, 1978.
29. Secker Walker LM, Sandler RM: Acute myeloid leukaemia with monosomy-7 follows acute lymphoblastic leukaemia. Br J Haematol 38:359-366, 1978.
30. Hutter JJ, Hays T, Rosen RC, Shende A, Lanzkowsky P, Corrigan JJ: Myelogenous leukemia evolving during the course of lymphoid malignancy in children. Am J Hematol 6:333-341, 1979.
31. Spector G, Youness E, Culbert SJ: Acute lymphoblastic leukemia followed by acute granulocytic leukemia in a pediatric patient. Am J Clin Pathol 72:242-245, 1979.

32. Miller DR, Leikin S, Albo V, Vitale L, Sather H, Coccia P, Nesbit M, Karon M, Hammond D: Use of prognostic factors in improving the design and efficiency of clinical trials in childhood leukemia: Children's cancer study group report. Cancer Treat Rep 64:381–392, 1980.

33. Chessels JM, Hardisty RM, Rapson NT, Greaves MF: Acute lymphoblastic leukemia in children: Classification and prognosis. Lancet 2:1307–1309, 1977.

34. Cimino MC, Rowley JD, Kinnealey A, Variakojis D, Golomb HM: Banding studies of chromosomal abnormalities in patients with acute lymphocytic leukemia. Cancer Res 39:227–238, 1979.

35. Kaneko Y, Rowley JD, Variakojis D, Chilcote RR, Check I and Sakurai M: Correlation of karyotype with clinical features in acute lymphoblastic leukemia (ALL). Cancer Res. (in press).

36. Slater RM, Philip P, Badsberg E, Behrendt H, Hansen NE, van Heerde P: A 14q+ chromosome in a B-cell acute lymphocytic leukemia and in a leukemic non-endemic Burkitt lymphoma. Int J Cancer 23:639–647, 1979.

37. Mitelman F, Anvret-Andersson M, Brandt L, Catovsky D, Klein G, Manolov G, Manolova Y, Mark-Vendel E, Nilsson PG: Reciprocal 8;14 translocation in EBV-negative B-cell acute lymphocytic leukemia with Burkitt-type cells. Int J Cancer 24:27–33, 1979.

38. Berger R, Bernheim A, Flandrin G, Daniel M-T, Schaison G, Brovet J-C, Bernard J: Translocation t(8;14) dans la leucémie lymphoblastique de type Burkitt. Nouv Presse Med 8:181–183, 1979.

39. Kaneko Y, Rowley JD, Check I, Variakojis D, Moohr JW: The 14q+ chromosome in pre-B-ALL. Blood 56:782–785, 1980.

40. Miyoshi I, Hiraki S, Kimura I, Miyamoto K, Sato J: 2/8 translocation in a Japanese Burkitt's lymphoma. Experientia 35:742, 1979.

41. Berger R, Bernheim A, Weh H-J, Flandrin G, Daniel MT, Brouet J-C, Colbert N: A new translocation in Burkitt's tumor cells. Human Genetics 53:111–112, 1979.

42. Rowley JD, Variakojis D, Kaneko Y, Cimino M: A Burkitt-lymphoma variant translocation (2p−;8q+) in a patient with ALL, L₃ (Burkitt type). Human Genet 58:166–167, 1981.

43. Van den Berghe H, David G, Broeckaert-Van Orshoven A, Louwagie A, Verwilghen R, Casteels-Van Daele M, Eggermont E, Eeckels R: A new chromosome anomaly in acute lymphoblastic leukemia (ALL). Hum Genet 46:173–180, 1979.

44. Kessous A, Corberand J, Grozdea J, Colombies P: Clone cellulaire à 27 chromosomes dans une leucémie aigue humaine. Nouv Rev Fr Hematol 15:73–82, 1975.

45. Oshimura M, Freeman AI, Sandberg AA: Chromosomes and causation of human cancer and leukemia. XXIII. Near-haploidy in acute leukemia. Cancer 40:1143–1148, 1977.

46. Prieto F, Badia L, Mayans J, Gomis F, Marty ML: Hipodiploidia de 26 cromosomas en leucemia linfoblastica aguda. Sangre 23:484–488, 1978.

47. Shabtai F, Lewinski UH, Har-Zahav L, Gaffer U, Halbrecht I, Djaldetti M: Haploidy in stem cell leukemia. Am J Clin Pathol 72:1018–1024, 1979.

48. Kaneko Y, Sakurai M: Acute lymphocytic leukemia (ALL) with near-haploidy—A unique group of ALL? Cancer Genet Cytogenet 2:13–18, 1980.

49. Secker Walker LM, Lawler SD, Hardisty RM: Prognostic implications of chromosomal findings in acute lymphoblastic leukaemia at diagnosis. Br Med J 2:1529–1530, 1978.

50. Kaneko Y, Hayashi Y, Sakurai M: Chromosomal findings and their correlation to prognosis in acute lymphocytic leukemia. Cancer Genet Cytogenet 4:227–235, 1981.

51. Third International Workshop on Chromosomes in Leukemia. Cancer Genet Cytogenet 4: 95–142, 1981.

52. Whang-Peng J, Knutsen T, Ziegler J, Leventhal B: Cytogenetic studies in acute lymphocytic leukemia: Special emphasis in long-term survival. Med Pediatr Oncol 2:333–351, 1976.

53. Zech L, Hoglund U, Nilsson K, Klein G: Characteristic chromosomal abnormalities in biopsies and lymphoid-cell lines from patients with Burkitt and non-Burkitt lymphomas. Int J Cancer 17:47–56, 1976.
54. Kaiser-McCaw B, Epstein AL, Kaplan HL, Hecht F: Chromosome 14 translocation in African and North American Burkitt's lymphoma. Int J Cancer 19:482–486, 1977.
55. First International Workshop on Chromosomes in Leukaemia. Chromosomes in Ph[1]-positive chronic granulocytic leukaemia. Br J Haematol 39:305–309, 1978.
56. Rowley JD, Fukuhara S: Chromosome studies in non-Hodgkin's lymphomas. Semin Oncol 7:255–266, 1980.
57. Daniel A, Francis SE, Stewart LA, Barber S: A near-haploid clone: 24,XY,t(9;22)(q34;q11) from a patient in blast crisis of chronic myeloid leukaemia. Scand J Haematol 21:99–103, 1978.
58. Hartley SE, Cook MK: Near-haploidy in a case of chronic myeloid leukemia. Cancer Genet Cytogenet 1:169–176, 1979.
59. Como RM, Graze PR: Emergence of a cell line with extreme hypodiploidy in blast crisis of chronic myelocytic leukemia. Blood 53:707–711, 1979.
60. Kessous A, Colombies P, Pris J, Clement D: Near-haploid cell line in lymphoid blast crisis of Ph[1]-positive chronic myeloid leukemia. Cancer Res 40:1354–1359, 1980.
61. Chessells JM, Janossy G, Lawler SD, Secker Walker LM: The Ph[1] chromosome in childhood leukaemia. Br J Haematol 41:25–41, 1979.
62. Bloomfield CD, Lingquist LL, Brunning RD, Yunis JJ, Coccia PF: The Philadelphia chromosome in acute leukemia. Virchow's Arch B Cell Pathol 29:81–92, 1978.
63. Whang-Peng J, Canellos GP, Carbone PP, Tjio JH: Clinical implications of cytogenetic variants in chronic myelocytic leukemia (CML). Blood 32:755–766, 1968.
64. Hagemeijer A, Van Zanen GE, Smit EME, Hahlen K: Bone marrow karyotypes of children with nonlymphocytic leukemia. Pediatr Res 13:1247–1254, 1979.
65. Hays T, Morse H, Peakman D, Rose B, Robinson A: Cytogenetic studies of chronic myelocytic leukemia in children and adolescents. Cancer 44:210–214, 1979.
66. Rowley JD: Unpublished data.
67. Boggs DR: Hematopoeitic stem cell theory in relation to possible lymphoblastic conversion of chronic myeloid leukemia. Blood 44:449–453, 1974.
68. Mauri C, Torelli U, di Prisco U, Silingardi V, Artusi T, Emilia G: Lymphoid blastic crisis at the onset of chronic granulocytic leukemia. Cancer 40:865–870, 1977.
69. Sandberg AA, Kohno S, Wake N, Minowada J: Chromosomes and causation of human cancer and leukemia. XLII. Ph[1]-positive ALL: An entity within myeloproliferative disorders? Cancer Genet Cytogenet 2:145–174, 1980.
70. Catovsky D: Ph[1]-positive acute leukaemia and chronic granulocytic leukaemia: One or two diseases? Br J Haematol 42:493–498, 1979.
71. Smith KL, Johnson W: Classification of chronic myelocytic leukemia in children. Cancer 34:670–679, 1974.
72. Altman AJ, Palmer CG, Baehner RL: Juvenile 'chronic granulocytic' leukaemia: A panmyelopathy with prominent monocytic involvement and circulating monocyte colony-forming cells. Blood 43:341–350, 1974.
73. Inoue S, Ravindranath Y, Thompson RI, Zuelzer WW, Ottenbreit MJ: Cytogenetics of juvenile type chronic granulocytic leukemia. Cancer 39:2017–2024, 1977.
74. Brodeur GM, Dow LW, Williams DL: Cytogenetic features of juvenile chronic myelogenous leukemia. Blood 53:812–819, 1979.
75. Miller RW: Persons with exceptionally high risk of leukemia. Cancer Res 27:2420–2423, 1967.
76. Engel RR, Hammond D, Eitzman DV, Pearson H, Krivit W: Transient congenital leukemia in 7 infants with mongolism. J Pediatr 65:303–305, 1964.

78

77. Ross JD, Molony WC, Desforges JF: Ineffective regulation of granulopoiesis masquerading as congenital leukemia in a mongoloid child. J Pediatr 63:1–10, 1963.
78. Brodeur GM, Dahl GV, Williams DL, Tipton RE, Kalwinsky DK: Transient leukemoid reaction and trisomy 21 mosaicism in a phenotypically normal newborn. Blood 55:691–693, 1980.
79. Kaneko Y, Rowley JD, Variakojis D, Chilcote RR, Moohr JW, Patel D: Chromosome abnormalities in Down's syndrome patients with acute leukemia. Blood 58:459–466, 1981.
80. Sakurai M, Sandberg AA: Prognosis of acute myeloblastic leukemia: Chromosomal correlation. Blood 41:93–104, 1973.
81. Nilsson PG, Brandt L, Mitelman F: Prognostic implication of chromosome analysis in acute non-lymphocytic leukemia. Leukemia Res 1:31–34, 1977.
82. Golomb HM, Vardiman JW, Rowley JD, Testa JR, Mintz U: Correlation of clinical findings with quinacrine-banded chromosomes in 90 adults with acute non-lymphocytic leukemia. N Engl J Med 299:613–619, 1978.
83. First International Workshop on Chromosomes in Leukaemia. Chromosomes in acute non-lymphocytic leukaemia. Br J Haematol 39:311–316, 1978.
84. Berger R, Bernheim A, Flandrin G: Hématologie. Absence d'anomalie chromosomique et leucémie aigue: Relations avec les cellules médullaires normales. C R Acad Sc Paris 290:1557–1559, 1980.

II. Pancreatic Malignancies

5. Genetic Aspects of Endocrine Neoplasia

R. NEIL SCHIMKE

Endocrine tumors in children are not common; hence, very little is known about their pathogenesis. The great bulk are probably environmentally induced like their adult counterparts. A few occur as components of certain heritable syndromes where the basic gene mutation presumably directly predisposes to tumor formation. This latter assumption is probably unprovable since a remote secondary rather than a pleiotropic effect of the gene may actually promote tumor development. It does appear, however, that whether primary or secondary, some mutant genes do render their possessor unusually susceptible to malignancy, and this susceptibility behaves as a mendelizing trait with varying degrees of penetrance and expressivity depending upon the gene in question. The topic has been reviewed in some detail [1].

1. GENES AND CANCER

Probably the best studies relating defective gene action to cancer have been accomplished in children with embryonal neoplasms [2]. These studies have also established that the same tumor can arise via different genetic mechanisms. For example, both a single gene defect and a chromosome deletion may predipsose to retinoblastoma. The precise molecular mechanism whereby cancer is initiated is rarely apparent with a few notable exceptions. One of them is xeroderma pigmentosa, where the gene mutation is associated with defective repair of ultraviolet light-induced damage to DNA [3]. A causal relationship between this defect and the skin cancer that eventually proves lethal in affected individuals is easy to visualize. It is less easy to explain heritable retinoblastoma which is generally considered to be a tissue-specific neoplasm. The issue is compounded even further by the

G. B. Humphrey et al. (eds.), Pancreatic Tumors in Children.
© *1982 Martinus Nijhoff Publishers, The Hague/Boston/London.* ISBN-13:978-94-009-7617-7

need to account for altered penetrance and expressivity even in affected families.

Probably the most generally accepted theory of hereditary oncogenesis has been proposed by Knudson and his colleagues [4]. They have suggested that the development of any malignancy requires at least two mutations, which could be of any type including a single gene change, a chromosome rearrangement or an environmental event. With heritable tumors, the initial mutation is assumed to be germinal, the second somatic. As a consequence of this sequence, inherited tumors would be more likely multifocal (or bilateral where paired organs are involved) and have an earlier average age of onset. Thus, decreased penetrance and incomplete monozygotic twin concordance could be explained by the lack of the second somatic mutation in a genetically predisposed host. Nonfamilial tumors would be most often, if not invariably, unifocal and appear somewhat later, since two independent somatic events would be required. Variable expressivity, e.g., individuals with either uni- or bilateral involvement in a family with heritable retinoblastoma could be accounted for by a reduced exposure of one eye to the environmental mutagen. This 'two-hit' model has been criticized on theoretical grounds, since it assumes that carcinogenesis is related to discrete, random mutational alterations that occur at a constant average rate, a phenomenon that may not be true [5]. Some prefer a three-hit model [6]. Alternative approaches have invoked variable host resistance [7], unstable [8], or delayed mutation [9], and defective regulatory genes [10]. The Knudson hypothesis may or may not ultimately be proved correct.

2. GENETICS AND ENDOCRINE TUMORS

The role genetic factors play in the pathogenesis of endocrine tumors exclusive of the multiple endocrine neoplasia (MEN) syndromes is variable, depending upon the individual gland. It is best to consider the evidence for each one separately.

2.1. Pituitary Tumors

The most common form of pituitary tumor in childhood and adolescence is a craniopharyngioma, a tumor derived from remnants of Rathke's pouch. It comprises about 10% of all intracranial tumors in children and is the most frequent subtentorial mass tumor in this age group [11, 12]. There is no evidence for genetic factors in its etiology.

Functional pituitary tumors in children are far less common. The only evidence for a heritable form, and that in older individuals, is provided by a few familial examples of acromegaly, most of which are in the preradioimmunoassay era and are thus not verifiable [13]. Levin et al. recorded 21-

and 20-year old brothers [14]. The younger brother had excessive growth early, then developed acromegaly, the older had only acromegaly. Both had acanthosis nigricans. A mother-daughter pair with tumors and the amenorrhea-galactorrhea syndrome has been recorded [15]. Fisch *et al.* described an acromegalic mother who delivered an infant with bony synostoses, large size and accelerated bone age [16]. The child's growth subsequently normalized. It is not likely HGH crossed the placenta, but perhaps certain growth factors such as one or more of the somatomedins could have accounted for the neonatal findings. It is important to exclude the diagnosis of cerebral gigantism (Soto syndrome) and pachydermoperiostosis, since these irregular dominant disorders may mimic pituitary gigantism in children.

Cushing's syndrome on a hypothalamic-lituitary basis is virtually never familial either in children or adults. Thyrotropin and gonadatropin-producing tumors are quite rare and also are not familial. Pituitary microadenomas have been reported in a few adult patients with the Turner and Klinefelter syndrome, presumably on the basis of long-term absent negative central feedback [17]. Isosexual precocity in children is generally hypothalamic and nontumorous with females being the most commonly affected sex. Male isosexual precocity does occur and can be heritable, but again it can not be related in most instances to endocrine neoplasia [18].

2.2. Thyroid

The incidence of thyroid cancer has increased in the United States over the past 25 years [19]. This increase has largely been attributed to late effects of external irradiation administered in childhood generally for benign disease. The post-irradiation risk in one study has been estimated at about 7% [20]. More recently, thyroid carcinoma has been seen after therapeutic irradiation for childhood neoplasms such as medulloblastoma [21] and cervical neuroblastoma [22]. There is no evidence that either diagnostic or therapeutic radioiodine in adults is carcinogenic. Whether the diagnostic use of I^{131} is carcinogenic in children remains controversial. The incidence of carcinoma is higher in young thyrotoxic patients treated with therapeutic radioiodine [23], but the doses used are smaller than in adults, and there is some evidence to suggest that were the amount given large enough to ablate the gland as is frequently the case in older individuals, this cancer risk could be avoided [24]. In all instances of childhood irradiation whether internal or external there is a 15-30-year latent period before the thyroid tumor develops. Thus, while the inciting event may occur in childhood, radiation-induced thyroid cancer is not a children's tumor. In fact, nonmedullary thyroid cancer in general is rare in children, with an incidence estimated at about one-twentieth of that in adults [25]. The tumor type is almost always papillary, follicular or mixed and only rarely anaplastic.

Save for medullary thyroid cancer (MTC), there is very little evidence for a specific genetic form of thyroid cancer. Papillary tumors have been reported in MEN I, and of course, MTC is invariable in MEN II and III but only in the latter disorder does it appear in children. MTC, which constitutes about 10% of all thyroid neoplasms, has also been recorded in families who show no evidence of other endocrinopathy and it is possible a pure form of heritable MTC exists independent of the MEN syndromes, although here again, the tumor does not occur in children [26]. There are a few rare families in which more than one individual has been affected with nonmedullary carcinoma. An affected father and his 12-year old daughter have been described [27]. The girl received external irradiation at age 4, and there was a family history of goiter on the father's side of the family. Similarly, two brothers with papillary carcinoma both had repeated chest fluoroscopy in childhood [28]. A mother with follicular carcinoma and her 9-year old son with a mixed tumor have been reported [29]. Two Norwegian families have been described in which 7 and 4 cases, respectively, of papillary carcinoma were found [30]. Although the youngest affected member was 17, the average age of the other patients was lower than a control group with a similar tumor. It is interesting that the background incidence of papillary carcinoma is comparatively high in that area of Norway. The authors cautiously suggested a possible relationship among atmospheric atomic tests, elevated I^{131} levels in milk and seafood some 20 years previously, and genetic factors. In the latter context, it is interesting that at least two other family members had cancer, a renal cell carcinoma in one and a glioblastoma in the other. These findings are reminiscent of those encountered in the cancer family syndrome where the risk of neoplasia behaves for practical purposes like an autosomal dominant trait [1]. In at least one type of cancer family, endocrine neoplasia, particularly of the adrenal and thyroid, does seem to be more frequent. Other family members suffer from embryonal neoplasms, brain tumors and acute leukemia, the latter in both children and adults, and breast carcinoma in women. Perhaps the kindreds with nonmedullary thyroid carcinoma actually have the cancer family syndrome, and as such have a genetic predilection to tumor formation, the type that surfaces being dependent upon the nature of the 'second hit' which in this instance could be excessive environmental radioiodine.

There are a number of genetic syndromes in which thyroid carcinoma has been described including certain inborn errors of thyroxine biosynthesis, and the Gardner, Cowden and Werner syndromes [2]. In these syndromes, the thyroid apparently shares in the generalized malignant diathesis conferred by the basic gene defect, since all three conditions are associated with neoplasms in a variety of tissues, the Gardner syndrome perhaps being the most malignant of the three. Cellular atypia is regularly seen in congenital goiters from patients with heritable defects in thyroxine biosynthesis, but frank tumor is relatively uncommon except in the Pendred syndrome, a condition in which goiter, due to some type of unidentified organification block is associated with sensorineural deafness [31], and in a newly described entity where follicular carcinoma developed in patients suffering from congenital goiter secondary to a persistent leak of nonhormonal iodide from the thyroid gland [32]. In both instances, prolonged, excessive TSH stimulation has been implicated in the pathogenesis of the carcinomas. In none of the foregoing disorders do thyroid tumors develop in children and in any case, the inheritance pattern is that of the primary syndrome.

2.3. Parathyroid Glands

It is difficult to estimate the proportion of cases of hyperparathyroidism that occur on a familial basis. About 85% are due to solitary adenomas, generally in females over the age of 40, and there is no evidence at all that these are due to heritable factors [33]. Diffuse hyperplasia of all glands occurs in the bulk of patients with MEN I and probably in more than a quarter of those with MEN II. When diffuse hyperplasia is found, it is likely that genetic factors are operational but no systematic studies have been undertaken in this regard. Christensson evaluated 16,000 people in Sweden between the ages of 20 and 63 and found 82 with hyperparathyroidism, only two of whom had a positive family history of the condition [34]. This figure is undoubtedly a gross underestimate of the familial incidence, since many affected individuals are totally asymptomatic. When hyperparathyroidism occurs in a family setting it is transmitted as an autosomal dominant trait. A number of workers feel that these families actually represent one of the MEN syndromes, the other endocrine glands simply not having shown any demonstrable evidence of hyperfunction at the time of study [35]. This interpretation may be an oversimplification since inherited tumors of other endocrine glands clearly exist outside the diagnostic confines of the MEN syndromes; e.g., pheochromocytoma, and independent hereditary hyperparathyroidism likely also exists.

The condition is uncommon in children, and even more rare in the neonatal period. Hillman *et al.* described sibs affected with neonatal hyperparathyroidism who were the offspring of a consanguineous union [36]. However, later studies on the relatives of such children revealed that they, too, were affected, indicating that a neonatal onset is just one age extreme of hereditary hyperparathyroidism [37]. In children, hyperparathyroidism must be differentiated from hypercalcemia due to transient idiopathic hypercalcemia of infancy, familial hypocalciuric hypercalcemia (also termed benign hypercalcemia), hypervitaminosis D and a host of other conditions that are in the aggregate much more common.

External irradiation has been suggested as a cause of single parathyroid adenomas, just as for thyroid carcinoma [38]. In fact, parathyroid adenomas and papillary/follicular thyroid carcinomas are found together more often than expected by chance [39]. The thyroid tumor is usually asymptomatic and is discovered at neck exploration for hyperparathyroidism. Whether radiation can be blamed for the parathyroid tumors is open to question [40]. One might expect more parathyroid carcinomas under these circumstances, but reports of such have not been forthcoming. True carcinoma of the parathyroids is exceedingly rare, and this is only one report of a familial occurrence in a 20-year old man and his 33-year old sister [41].

Interestingly, small almost invariably single foci of MTC have been found on occasion in sporadic hyperparathyroidism [42]. Either these patients represent new MEN II mutations or they demonstrate that hypercalcemia of any cause, if persistent, can cause C-cell hyperplasia and, on occasion, MTC. Other nonendocrine tumors seem to be unduly frequent in patients with hyperparathyroidism with some series reporting a 30–40% coincidence [43]. The reasons for this are quite obscure, but it may be at least in part related to the fact that both parathyroid adenomas and cancer in general tend to develop in older individuals.

2.4. Adrenal Cortex

More than 80% of the time hyperfunction of the adrenal cortex in adults is due to excessive ACTH, either from the pituitary or from ectopic sources [44]. In contrast, primary adrenal disease predominates in children, with carcinoma being the tumor type in 65% of patients younger than age 15, the majority of whom are affected before the age of five [45]. Whereas Cushing's syndrome results from adrenal adenomas or carcinomas in adults, children are more likely to present with virilization [46, 47]. Feminization is relatively uncommon at any age [48]. The exact frequency of aldosteronomas is difficult to estimate, since it may vary depending upon the type of study, i.e., whether a normal or a hypertensive population is evaluated or whether the pathology is taken from a random surgical or autopsy series or from a group of hypertensive individuals. Aldosterone-producing tumors in children are rare no matter what the source of the patient material.

Adrenal-cortical tumors in adults have been described as part of MEN I, however, even in this disorder, the signs and symptoms of Cushing's syndrome are more commonly due to pituitary or ectopic ACTH rather than primary adrenal adenomatosis. Similarly, Cushing's syndrome in MEN II is due to ectopic ACTH, generally from the MTC. Adrenal-cortical tumors have been seen in the Gardner and Werner syndromes, again in old individuals. Familial Cushing's syndrome has been confined to two reports. In one Cuban family, three sibs, ages 13, 15 and 32, had adrenal-cortical hyperplasie, while a fourth, a 15-year old girl, had a virilizing adrenal carcinoma [49]. In the other family two of four sibs had the Cushing syndrome [50]. In both instances, the pathology in the adrenal was that of so-called microadenomatosis or primary nodular dysplasia. Interestingly, one of the affected sibs in the second family also carried a diagnosis of von Recklinghausen's disease, although there was no one else in the family known to be affected. Perhaps this form of adrenal disease is simply inherited, the two pedigrees suggesting autosomal recessive transmission.

Save for these reports there is no clear-cut evidence that a simple heritable form of adrenal carcinoma exists. Some earlier reports refer to tumors in sibs with congenital adrenal hyperplasia. While the adrenals in untreated cases can look histologically quite bizarre and even malignant, probably due to continuous ACTH stimulation [8], there is no firm evidence that any of these 'tumors' actually behaved in a malignant, i.e., metastatic, fashion [51]. On the other hand, as pointed out by Miller, there are some peculiarities in the occurrence of adrenal-cortical carcinomas in children [52]. For example, a rather significant array of second neoplasms has been reported in survivors, including brain tumors, rhabdomyosarcomas and osteosarcomas [53]. A family history of breast carcinoma or acute leukemia may be present. On occasion, the same tumor types may be seen in different individuals, e.g., adrenal carcinoma in one sib and brain tumor in another [54]. Adrenal-cortical carcinoma has been described in sibs on two occasions [55, 56]. In one of these families, the mother of the two affected sibs developed bilateral breast carcinoma and subsequently expired of an astrocytoma. These findings are compatible with one form of the cancer family syndrome. Thus, while adrenal-cortical carcinoma *per se* may not be inherited, at least a subset of such individuals may be at increased risk for second neoplasms and their relatives may be at equal risk for the same sort of tumors. The family history may be exceedingly important in differentiating the sporadic from the possibly familial case.

There are two other conditions that also seem to predispose to adrenal carcinoma in children. One of these, the Beckwith-Wiedemann syndrome, will be discussed later in relationship to neonatal hypoglycemia. The other is hemihypertrophy, an aberrant growth process that also predisposes to the development of Wilms' tumor and hepatoblastoma [57]. Hemihypertrophy is of course variable, and mostly it has been ascertained after discovery of a tumor, so that data are somewhat biased. The absolute risk for cancer given a child with hemihypertrophy is probably low.

The contemporary treatment for central Cushing's syndrome is a transsphenoidal pituitary microsurgery although bilateral adrenalectomy might still be appropriate in selected instances [58]. Rare cases may respond to cyproheptidine [59]. Adrenal carcinomas are often metastatic when diagnosed initially and require cytotoxic therapy [60].

2.5. Adrenal Medulla

Pheochromocytomas may be found at virtually any site where chromaffin cells exist, but more than 90% are located below the diaphragmn in or adjacent to the adrenal glands, the para-aortic area, the organ of Zuckerkandl or even in the urinary bladder [61]. The prevalence of the tumor has been estimated at 0.5–1/1000 in a random population, but this figure may be revised upward 5–6-fold in a hypertensive population [62]. Both sexes may be affected and the tumor has been found in all age groups, although it is 8–10 times more common in adults. The signs and symptoms are well known and need not be recounted. Only about 5% are asymptomatic. Occasionally, the tumors secrete ectopic peptides such as ACTH, PTH, calcitonin and VIP leading to diagnostic difficulties.

Exactly what proportion of pheochromocytomas is familial is difficult to assess, since some patients may have asymptomatic relatives or relatives destined to develop the tumor later in life. One study of 507 patients found 5% that were familial [63]. Theoretical consideratios led Knudsen and Strong to postulate that about 25% were familial [64]. As is generally the rule, familial tumors appear about 20 years earlier on the average, and they tend to be bilateral and/or multifocal. In some instances patients with unilateral tumors may develop second tumors months to years later. Children are particularly prone to have multiple, extra-adrenal lesions, and in the above context such children should be considered as having familial disease [65]. In one personally observed family, a 10-year old child was found to have a renal and para-aortic pheochromocytoma. His maternal grandfather and great-aunt both had had malignant pheochromocytomas of the organ of Zuckerkandl described in a report appearing 20 years ago [66]. The child's mother, brother and uncle have no current evidence of disease. Familial pheochromocytoma is inherited as an autosomal dominant trait, but as illustrated in the above family, penetrance is incomplete, probably being no greater than 90% by age 50. Malignant degeneration occurs in 5–10% of patients but may be quite difficult to diagnose, since distinction between primary multifocal and metastatic disease may not be easy [67].

Pheochromocytoma is an integral feature of MEN II and III. Perhaps as many as 5% of patients with von Recklinghausen's disease may develop pheochromocytomas. It also occurs in the von Hippel-Lindau syndrome and with islet cell carcinomas of the pancreas. While these conditions all show some common features, they are genetically distinct. In none of these latter conditions have pheochromocytomas appeared or at least been diagnosed in childhood. Nonetheless, it would be important to evaluate all first degree relatives of a child with pheochromocytoma, particularly if the tumor is multiple, looking for evidence of other affected individuals or for signs of these various syndromes.

Extra-adrenal pheochromocytomas are, technically speaking, paragangliomas, but this term is generally reserved for tumors of chemoreceptor tissue or chemodectomas. Paragangliomas are often histologically subdivided into chromaffin and nonchromaffin types or are separated on the basis of their ability to secrete catecholamines, but this distinction is considered by some to be artifactual [68]. Familial chemodectomas have been reported in an autosomal dominant inheritance pattern [69], but mixed families have also been described in which various members had either or both chemodectomas and pheochromocytomas [70]. In one such instance, a patient developed an adrenal pheochromocytoma, a paraganglioma and bilateral carotid body tumors at ages 11, 13 and 36 respectively [71]. While no convincingly environmental process is known to promote development of a pheochromocytoma, the appearance of a chemodectoma may be triggered by chronic hypoxia or hypercarbia [72]. True tumors of chemoreceptor organs are quite uncommon in children and when found, should alert one to seek a possible genetic basis.

2.6. Endocrine Pancreas

Hypoglycemia in the pediatric age range is moderately common. It may be due to a variety of factors, many of which have little to do with beta-cell function [73]. Hyperinsulinemia as a cause is a well-recognized complication of maternal diabetes mellitus, but it also is a reported complication of erythroblastosis for reasons not entirely clear. Islet cell adenomas producing excess insulin develop at any age, are usually single and are readily cured by simple excision. Save for those associated with MEN I which appear characteristically in adult life, the adenomas are not generally familial. There is only a single report in the literature of such an occurrence, a father and daughter each with islet cell adenomatosis [74].

A more unusual condition which may easily mimic an islet cell adenoma is nesidioblastosis, a term that refers to the pathologic finding of diffuse proliferation of disordered islet cells of all types throughout the pancreas [75]. The condition, when it occurs in the neonate is familial and the interpretation of the reported pedigrees is that it is an autosomal recessive trait [76, 77]. The basic lesion appears to reside in the failure of primitive islet cells to regress appropriately during embryonic life. Partial to complete pancreatotomy is usually necessary to control the severe, persistent hypoglycemia. Either nedisioblastosis or true beta-cell hyperplasia may be seen in the Beckwith-Wiedemann syndrome, a condition marked by generalized overgrowth of a variety of tissues with an increased incidence of embryonal malignancies [78]. The inheritance pattern of the syndrome has not been well worked out, although current evidence suggests it is an autosomal dominant trait with decreased penetrance [79].

As previously mentioned, the Z-E syndrome occurs in children but it has not been shown to be either familial or part of the MEN I spectrum in young individuals. Other islet cell tumors such as glucagonomas and somatostatinomas have not been reported in children. The typical patient with glucagonoma has diabetes mellitus, weight loss, stomatitis and a rather peculiar skin lesion, termed necrolytic migratory erythema. A recent survey of 42 cases noted that the tumor was nearly four times more common in women and was highly malignant, being commonly metastatic at the time of discovery [80]. Streptozotocin has been used therapeutically with inconsistent success. A new agent, dimethyltriazenoimidazole carboxamide shows some promise when resectability is impossible [81]. Glucagonoma may be an occasional part of MEN I.

Hyperglucagonemia has been reported as an independent autosomal dominant trait, having been found in multiple asymptomatic members of the family of a proband with an islet cell tumor [82]. Whether all these individuals had tumors or not is unknown. Patients with glucagonomas may only develop symptoms if the size of the glucagon molecule secreted is appropriate. Palmer et al. reported a kindred in which 9 of 15 members had elevated circulating levels of high molecular weight glucagon [83]. They postulated a defect in cleavage of proglucagon to glucagon. None of the individuals was symptomatic.

Somatostatinomas are considerably more rare, only a few cases having been reported, all in adults [84]. The typical finding, if such can be said after a review of six cases, is of a patient with diabetes mellitus, steatorrhea, weight loss and cholelithiasis. Interestingly, in three of the six cases, the islet cell tumor also produced other hormones, ACTH in one and calcitonin in two. As indicated earlier, islet cells seem to be prone to secrete ectopic peptides, some of which are generally considered to be hypothalamic or pituitary in origin [85]. Somatostatin is not truly an ectopic peptide, however, as it seems to be a normal constituent of the pancreatic islets.

The pancreatic cholera syndrome when it occurs in children, is generally not pancreatic in origin, but is due to excessive VIP secretion by ganglioneuromas [86]. There is one recorded case of a 2-week old infant with secretory diarrhea who was found to have non-beta islet cell hyperplasia [87]. Such cases are extraordinarily rare.

2.7. Gonadal Tumors

Testicular tumors are diagnosed in less than 1/50,000 males. Most are of germ cell origin in adults, whereas in children teratomas and stromal tumors predominate. Gonadoblastomas contain both stromal and germ cell elements, but these tumors occur almost exclusively in the dysgenetic gonads of XY individuals, who usually have sexual ambiguity, or in individuals with sex chromosome mosaicism in whom a dysgenetic gonad contains a Y-chromosome cell line. Cryptorchidism also confers a 10–15-fold increased risk of malignancy [88].

Familial aggregation of testicular tumors has been reported, albeit infrequently. In adults, affected twins, nontwin subs and father–son constellations have been noted, although less than 50 of such instances have been recorded [89, 90]. Commensurate with a genetic etiology in these families is the general tendency for the tumors to be bilateral and for monozygotic twin concordance to be high. Ethnic differences also support a role for genetic factors. Most reports make no mention of family history or of other neoplasms in relatives save for that of Lynch *et al.* [91]. It is possible that a simply inherited form of testicular neoplasm exists but the data are so meager that no firm genetic conclusion can be recorded.

Testicular teratomas are usually but not invariably parthenogenetic in origin. Affected sibs have been described on two occasions, and in one instance the brothers had the Klinefelter syndrome [92, 93]. This latter observation is probably not a coincidence, since extragonadal teratomas or choriocarcinomas have been seen on a number of occasions in patients with an XXY karyotype [94–97]. They have been mostly located in the mediastinum but hypothalamic and retroperitoneal tumors have also been reported. A common presentation is sexual precocity due to excessive HCG secretion, and it is often this feature that leads to the chromosome evaluation and hence the diagnosis of the Klinefelter syndrome.

Ovarian carcinoma is roughly five times more frequent than testicular cancer. About 90% of the adult-onset tumors are derived from germinal epithelium, and they tend to occur in older women. Incidence rates vary around the world, and changing rates in migrant populations suggest a potent role for environmental factors, but nothing definite has been identified [98]. Alternatively, there are a number of reports of apparent multigeneration transmission of ovarian cancer [1]. Unlike the situation with most familial tumors, however, the neoplasms are most often unilateral, and the age of onset is generally similar to that seen in the nonfamilial cases. It is possible that 5–10% of ovarian neoplasms in adults are familial with the tendency to develop the tumors inherited as a sex-limited autosomal or an X-linked trait. Unfortunately, the generally late age of onset precludes good genetic studies.

Ovarian carcinomas may be part of the cancer family complex in which other family members develop adenocarcinomas of a variety of sites, i.e., breast and endometrium in females, stomach and prostate in males, and colon in both sexes [99]. This form of cancer family syndrome appears to be distinct from the other type in which various individuals develop embryonal neoplasms, sarcomas, and endocrine tumors not of the reproductive system.

Ovarian tumors in children and adolescents are only a small proportion of all ovarian neoplasms, one series citing a 6% incidence [100]. They are often histologically complex and classification is difficult. In a group of 353 tumors, Norris and Jensen identified 58% that were germ cell in origin, about two-thirds of which were malignant [100]. Epithelial and stromal tumors were about equally frequent, 19% and 18% respectively, and the remainder were either nonclassifiable or unusual, such as lymphomas. The bulk of the germ cell tumors were teratomas or contained teratomatous elements. These tumors may be familial, tend to be bilateral and curiously often undergo torsion [101]. Affected twins, triplets, sibs and a mother-daughter combination have been described, suggesting that there may be a rare form of dominantly inherited ovarian teratoma.

A two-generation family with dysgerminoma has been described [102]. Arrhenoblastomas have been reported in a family whose affected members also had thyroid adenomas [103]. Ovarian fibromas have been recorded in four generations of a family [104]. Granulosa cell tumors may develop in 10–20% of female patients with the Peutz-Jegher syndrome [1]. Ovarian tumors, usually but not invariably benign, have been described in the Gardner and basal cell nevus syndromes and in ataxia-telangiectasia [1]. These scattered reports do not allow for any meaningful interpretation of the proportion of ovarian neoplasms that might be familial. Clearly, systematic studies are necessary in this regard.

Gonadal neoplasms do not appear to develop in patients with abnormal sexual differentiation unless the gonad is dysgenetic and/or contains a Y-chromosome cell line [105]. Even then the risk is variable, ranging from zero in XX males with H-Y antigen-positive to 20–30% in patients with XO/XY mosaicism (mixed gonadal dysgenesis) or with the H-Y antigen positive form of XY pure gonadal dysgenesis. Gonadal malignancy has been documented, albeit rarely in true hermaphroditism [106]. With the complete form of testicular feminization, the risk is about 10%. There seems to be little risk with the incomplete forms, but such cases are relatively few in number. Inborn errors of steroid metabolism, whether gonadal or adrenal or both do not seem to predispose to malignancy in either sex. The testicular masses detected in males with virilizing adrenal hyperplasia generally regress with cortisol therapy and are therefore considered to be composed of hypertrophied adrenal rest tissue.

Save for the H-Y antigen-positive form of XY pure gonadal dysgenesis, malignancy in the gonads of children with intersex states has not been described. In this condition, prophylactic gonadectomy should be undertaken as soon as the diagnosis is made.

REFERENCES

1. Schimke RN: Genetics and Cancer in Man. Edinburgh: Churchill Livingston, 1978.
2. Schimke RN: Genetics and cancer in children: current concepts. In: Genetic Issues in Pediatrics and Gynecology, Kaback M (ed). New York: Year Book (in press).
3. Harnden DG, Taylor AM: Chromosomes and neoplasia. Adv Hum Genet 9:1-70; 355-360, 1979.
4. Knudson AG, Strong LC, Anderson DE: Heredity and cancer in man. Prog Med Genet 9:113-158, 1973.
5. Vogel F: Genetics of retinoblastoma. Hum Genet 52:1-54, 1979.
6. Bonaiti-Pellie C, Briard-Guillemot ML, Feingold J, Frezal J: Associated congenital malformations in retinoblastoma. Clin Genet 7(1):37-39, 1975.
7. Matsunaga E: Hereditary retinoblastoma: delayed mutation or host resistance? Am J Hum Genet 30:406-424, 1978.
8. Goudie RB: Unstable mutations in vitiligo, organ-specific autoimmune diseases, and multiple endocrine adenoma/peptic-ulcer syndrome. Lancet 2(8189):285-287, 1980.
9. Herrmann J: Delayed mutation as a cause of retinoblastoma; Application to Genetic Counseling. Birth Defects 12:79-90, 1976.
10. Comings DE: A general theory of carcinogenesis. Proc Natl Acad Sci (USA) 70:3324-3328, 1973.
11. Banna M, Hoarse RD, Stanley P, Till K: Craniopharyngioma in children. J Pediatr 83:781-785, 1973.
12. Thomsett MJ, Conte FA, Kaplan SL, Grumbach MM: Endocrine and neurologic outcome in childhood craniopharyngioma: review of effect of treatment in 42 patients. J Pediatr 97:728-735, 1980.
13. Koch G, Tiwisina T: Beitrag zur Erblichkeit der Akromegalie und der Hyperostosis generalisata mit Pachydermic. Arzt Forsch 13:489-504, 1959.
14. Levin SR, Hofeldt FO, Becker N, Wilson CB, Seymour R, Forsham PH: Hypersomatotropism and acanthosis nigricans in two brothers. Arch Intern Med 134:365-367, 1974.
15. Linquette M, Herlant M, Laine E, Fossati P, Dupont-Lecompte M: Adénome à prolactine chez une jeune fille dont la mère était porteuse d'un adenome hypophysaire avec anemorrhea-galactorrhée. Ann Endocrinol 28:773-780, 1967.
16. Fisch RO, Prem KA, Feinberg SB, Gehrz RC: Acromegaly in a gravida and her infant. Obstet Gynecol 43:861-866, 1974.
17. Samaan NA, Stepanas AV, Danziger J, Trujillo J: Reactive pituitary abnormalities in patients with Klinefelter's and Turner's syndromes. Arch Intern Med 139:198-201, 1979.
18. Jacobsen AW, Macklin MT: Hereditary sexual precocity: report of a family with 27 affected members. Pediatrics 9:682-695, 1952.
19. Weiss W: Changing incidence of thyroid cancer. J Nat Cancer Inst 62:1137-1142, 1979.
20. Roudebush CP, Asteris GT, DeGroot LJ: Natural history of radiation associated thyroid cancer. Arch Intern Med 138:1631-1634, 1978.

21. Roggli VL, Estrada R, Fechner RE: Thyroid neoplasm following irradiation for medullo-blastoma. Cancer 43:2232–2238, 1979.
22. McKenzie CG, Hope-Stone HF: Multiple adenomas of the thyroid occurring 20 years after successful radiotherapy for neuroblastomas in the cervical lymph nodes. Br J Radiol 48:1028–1031, 1975.
23. Dobyns BM, Sheline GE, Workman JB: Malignant and benign neoplasms of the thyroid in patients treated for hyperthyroidism: a report of the cooperative thyrotoxicosis therapy follow-up study. J Clin Endocrinol Metab 38:976–995, 1974.
24. Holm LE, Dahlqvist I, Israelsson A, Lundell G: Malignant thyroid tumors after iodine-131 therapy. N Engl J Med 303:188–191, 1980.
25. Joppich I, Roher HO, Hecker WC, Knorr D, Daum R: Besonderheiten des Schilddrüsen Karzinoms in Kindersalter. Klin Paediatr 192:436–439, 1980.
26. Hillyard CJ, Evans IM, Hill PA, Taylor S: Familial medullary thyroid carcinoma. Lancet 1(8072):1009–1011, 1978.
27. Lacour J, Vignalou J, Perez R, Gerard-Marchant R: Epithelioma papillaire du corps thyroide. Nouv Press Med 2:2249–2252, 1973.
28. Fisher C, Edmonds CJ: Papillary carcinoma of the thyroid in two brothers after chest fluoroscopy in childhood. Br Med J 281:1600–1601, 1980.
29. Nemec J, Soumar J, Zamrazll V, et al.: Familial occurrence of differentiated (non-medullary) thyroid cancer. Oncology 32:151–157, 1975.
30. Lote K, Andersen K, Nordel E: Familial occurrence of papillary thyroid carcinoma. Cancer 46:1291–1297, 1980.
31. Illum P: Thyroid carcinoma in Pendred's syndrome. J Laryngol Otol 92:435–439, 1978.
32. Cooper DS, Axelrod L, DeGroot LJ: Congenital goiter and the development of metastatic follicular carcinoma with evidence for a leak of nonhormonal iodide: chemical, pathological, kinetic, and biochemical studies and a review of the literature. J Clin Endocrinol Metab 52:294–306, 1981.
33. Muller H: Sex, age and hyperparathyroidism. Lancet 1:449–450, 1969.
34. Christensson T: Familial hyperparathyroidism. Ann Intern Med 85:614–615, 1976.
35. Jackson CE, Boonstra CE: The relationship of hereditary hyperparathyroidism to endocrine adenomatosis. Am J Med 43:727–734, 1967.
36. Hillman DA, Scriver CR, Pedvis S: Neonatal familial primary hyperparathyroidism. N Engl J Med 270:483–490, 1964.
37. Spiegel AM, Harrison HE, Marx SJ: Neonatal primary hyperparathyroidism with autosomal dominant inheritance. J Pediatr 90:269–272, 1977.
38. Russ JE, Scanlon EF, Sever SF: Parathyroid adenomas following irradiation. Cancer 43:1078–1083, 1979.
39. LiVolsi VA, LoGerfo P, Feind CR: Coexistent parathyroid adenomas and thyroid carcinoma: can radiation be blamed. Arch Surg 113:285–286, 1978.
40. LiVolsi VA, Feind CR: Parathyroid adenoma and nonmedullary thyroid carcinoma. Cancer 38:1391–1393, 1976.
41. Frayha RA, Nassar VH, Dagher F, Salti IS: Familial parathyroid carcinoma. Leb Med J 25:299–309, 1972.
42. LiVolsi VA, Feind CR: Incidental medullary thyroid carcinoma in sporadic hyperparathyroidism. Am J Clin Pathol 71:595–599, 1979.
43. Farr HW, Fahey TJ Jr, Nash AG: Primary hyperparathyroidism and cancer. Am J Surg 126:539–543, 1973.
44. Gold EM: The Cushing Syndrome: changing views of diagnosis and treatment. Ann Intern Med 90:829–844, 1979.
45. Gilbert MG, Cleveland WW: Cushing's syndrome in infancy. Pediatrics 46:217–229,

1970.

46. Benaily M, Schweisguth O, Job LC: Les tumeurs cortico-surrénales de l'infant. Arch Fr Pediatr 32:441–453, 1975.

47. King DR, Lack EE: Adrenal cortical carcinoma: a clinical and pathologic study of 49 cases. Cancer 44:239–244, 1979.

48. Zaitoon MM, Mackie GG: Adrenal cortical tumors in children. Urology 12:645–649, 1978.

49. Arce B, Licea M, Hung S, Padron R: Familial Cushing's syndrome. Acta Endocrinol 87:139–147, 1978.

50. Schweizer-Cagianut M, Froesch ER, Hedinger C: Familial Cushing's syndrome with primary adrenocortical microadenomatosis (primary adrenocortical nodular dysplasia). Acta Endocrinol 94:529–535, 1980.

51. Hain SM: Adrenal tumors and pseudohermaphroditism: a hormone study of cases. J Path Bact 59:267–292, 1947.

52. Miller RW: Peculiarities in the occurrence of adrenal cortical carcinoma. Am J Dis Child 132:235–236, 1978.

53. Meadows AT, D'Angio GJ, Mike V, Banfi A, Harris C, Jenkin RD, Schwartz A: Patterns of second malignant neoplasms in children. Cancer 40(4 suppl):1903–1911, 1977.

54. Draper GJ, Heaf MM, Kinnier Wilson LM: Occurrence of childhood cancers among sibs and estimation of familial risks. J Med Genet 14:81–90, 1977.

55. Mahloudji M, Ronaghy H, Dutz W: Virilizing adrenal carcinoma in two sibs. J Med Genet 8:160–163, 1971.

56. Rimoin DL, Schimke RN: Genetic Disorders of the Endocrine Glands. St Louis: CV Mosby, 1971, p 235.

57. Fraumeni JF Jr, Miller RW: Adreno-cortical neoplasms with hemihypertrophy, brain tumors and other disorders. J Pediatr 70:129–138, 1967.

58. Bigos ST, Somma M, Rasid E, Eastman RC, Lanthier A, Johnston HH, Hardy J: Cushing's disease: management by transsphenoidal pituitary microsurgery. J Clin Endocrinol Metab 50:348–354, 1980.

59. Grant DB, Atherden SM: Cushing's disease presenting with growth failure: clinical remission during cyproheptadine therapy. Arch Dis Child 54:466–468, 1979.

60. Hogan TF, Gilchrist KW, Westring DW, Citrin DL: A clinical and pathologic study of adrenocortical carcinoma: therapeutic implications. Cancer 45:2880–2883, 1980.

61. Melicow MM: One hundred cases of pheochromocytoma (107 tumors) at the Columbia-Presbyterian Medical Center 1926–1976: a clinicopathological analysis. Cancer 40:1987–2004, 1977.

62. DeQuattro V, Campese VM: Pheochromocytoma: diagnosis and therapy. In: Endocrinology, Vol 2, DeGroot LJ, Cahill GF Jr, Odell WD, Martin L, Potts JT Jr, Nelson DH, Steinberger E, Winegrad AI (eds). New York: Grune and Stratton, 1979, pp 1279–1288.

63. Herman H, Mornex R: Human tumors secreting catecholamines. New York: Macmillan Co, 1964.

64. Knudson AF Jr, Strong LC: Mutation and cancer: neuroblastoma and pheochromocytomas. Am J Hum Genet 24:514–532, 1972.

65. Stackpole RH, Melicow MM, Uson AC: Pheochromocytoma in children. J Pediatr 63:314–330, 1963.

66. Cook JE, Urich RW, Sample HG Jr, Fawcett NW: Peculiar familial and malignant pheochromocytomas of the organs of Zuckerkandl. Ann Intern Med 52:126–133, 1960.

67. Palmieri G, Ikkos D, Luft R: Malignant pheochromocytoma. Acta Endocrinol 36:549–560, 1961.

68. Schwartz EL, Mao P, Hernried P, Born EE, Waldamann EB: Catecholamine- secreting

paragaglioma. Arch Intern Med 135:978–985, 1975.

69. Grufferman S, Gillman MW, Pasternake LR, Peterson CL, Young WG Jr: Familial carotid body tumors. Cancer 46:2116–2122, 1980.

70. Pollack RS: Carotid body tumors—idiosyncracies. Oncology 27:81–91, 1973.

71. Revak CS, Morris SE, Alexander GH: Pheochromocytoma and recurrent chemodectomas over a twenty-five-year period. Radiology 100:53–54, 1971.

72. Chedid A, Jao W: Hereditary tumors of the carotid bodies and chronic obstructive pulmonary disease. Cancer 33:1635–1641, 1974.

73. Pagliara AS, Karl IE, Haymond M, Kipnis DM: Hypoglycemia in infancy and childhood. J Pediatr 82:365–379, 1973.

74. Tragl KH, Mayr WR: Familial islet-cell adenomatosis. Lancet 2:426–428, 1977.

75. Knight J, Garvin PJ, Danis RK, Lewis JE Jr, Willman VL: Nesidioblastosis in children. Arch Surg 115:880–882, 1980.

76. Schwartz SS, Rich BH, Lucky AW, Straus FH II, Gonen B, Wolfsdorf J, Thorp FW, Burrington JD, Madden JD, Rubenstein AH, Rosenfeld RL: Familial nesidioblastosis: severe neonatal hypoglycemia in two families. J Pediatr 95:44–53, 1979.

77. Hammersen G, Trefz FK: Familial nesidioblastosis. J Pediatr 96:778, 1980.

78. Sotelo-Avila C, Gooch WM III: Neoplasms associated with the Beckwith-Wiedemann syndrome. Perspect Pediatr Pathol 3:255–272, 1976.

79. Ben-Galim E, Gross-Kieselstein M, Abrahamov A: Beckwith-Wiedemann syndrome in a mother and her son. Am J Dis Child 131:801–803, 1977.

80. Leichter SB: Clinical and metabolic aspects of glucagonoma. Medicine 59:100–113, 1980.

81. Strauss GM, Weitzman SA, Aoki TT: Dimethyltriazenoimidazole carboxamide therapy of malignant glucagonoma. Ann Intern Med 90:57–58, 1979.

82. Boden G, Owen OE: Familial hyperglucagonemia — an autosomal dominant disorder. N Engl J Med 296:534–538, 1977.

83. Palmer JP, Werner PL, Benson JW, Ensink JW: Dominant inheritance of large molecular weight immunoreactive glucagon. J Clin Invest 61:763–769, 1978.

84. Krejs GJ, Orci L, Conlon JM, Ravazzola M, Davis GR, Raskin P, Collins SM, McCarthy DM, Baetens D, Rubinstein A, Aldor TA, Unger RH: Somatostatinoma syndrome. N Engl J Med 301:285–292, 1979.

85. Wahlstrom T, Seppala M: Luteinizing hormone-releasing factor-like immunoreactivity in islet cells and insulinomas of the human pancreas. Int J Cancer 24:744–748, 1979.

86. Kaplan SJ, Holbrook CT, McDaniel HG, Buntain WL, Crist WM: Vasoactive intestinal peptide secreting tumors of childhood. Am J Dis Child 134:21–24, 1980.

87. Ghishan FK, Soper RT, Nassif EG, Younoszai MK: Chronic diarrhea of infancy-non-beta islet cell hyperplasia. Pediatrics 64:46–49, 1978.

88. Simpson JL, Photopulos G: Hereditary aspects of ovarian and testicular neoplasia. Birth Defects 2:51–60, 1976.

89. Kademian MT, Caldwell WL: Testicular seminoma: a case report of two brothers with seminoma and a review of the literature of testicular malignancies occurring in closely related family members. J Urol 116:380–381, 1976.

90. Vaccari E: Testicular seminoma in father and son. Andrologia 11:250–254, 1979.

91. Lynch HT, Krush AJ, Mulcahy GM, Reed WB: Familial occurrence of a variety of premalignant diseases and uncommon malignant neoplasms. Cancer 33:1474–1479, 1974.

92. Shinohara M, Komatsu H, Kawamura T, Yokoyama M: Familial testicular teratoma in 2 children: familial report and review of the literature. J Urol 123:552–555, 1980.

93. Gustavson KH, Gamstorp I, Meueling S: Bilateral teratoma of the testes in two brothers with 47, XXY Klinefelter's syndrome. Clin Genet 8:5–10, 1975.

94. Floret D, Renaud H, Monnet P: Sexual precocity and thoracic polyembryoma: Klinefelter syndrome. J Pediatr 94:163, 1979.
95. Sogge MR, McDonald SD, Cofold PB: The malignant potential of the dysgenetic germ cell in Klinefelter's syndrome. Am J Med 66:515–518, 1979.
96. Chaussain JL, Lamerle J, Roger M, Canlorbe P, Job JC: Klinefelter syndrome, tumor, and sexual precocity. J Pediatr 97:607–609, 1980.
97. Weetman AP, Borysiewicz LK: Androgen production in a patient with Klinefelter's syndrome and choriocarcinoma. Br Med J 2:585–586, 1980.
98. Annegers JF, Strom H, Decker DG, Dockerty MB, O'Fallon WM: Ovarian cancer. Cancer 43:723–729, 1979.
99. Lynch HT, Lynch PM: Tumor variation in the cancer family syndrome: ovarian cancer. Am J Surg 138:439–442, 1979.
100. Norris HJ, Jensen RD: Relative frequency of ovarian neoplasms in children and adolescents. Cancer 30:713–719, 1972.
101. Brown EH Jr: Identical twins with twisted benign cystic teratoma of the ovary. Am J Obstet Gynecol 134:879–880, 1979.
102. Jackson SM: Ovarian dysgerminoma in three generations? J Med Genet 4:112–113, 1967.
103. Jensen RD, Norris HJ, Fraumeni JF Jr: Familial arrhenoblastoma and thyroid adenoma. Cancer 33:218–223, 1974.
104. Dumont-Herskowitz RA, Safari HS, Senior B: Ovarian fibromata in four successive generations. J Pediatr 93:621–624, 1978.
105. Simpson JL, Photopulos G: The relationship of neoplasia to disorders of abnormal sexual differentiation. Birth Defects 12:15–50, 1976.
106. Radharrishnan S, Sivaraman L, Natarajan PS: True hermaphrodite with multiple gonadal neoplasms: report of a case with cytogenetic study. Cancer 42:2726–2732, 1978.

6. Tumors of the Exocrine Pancreas in Childhood

Tumors of nonendocrine pancreatic epithelium are rare to very rare in infancy and childhood. In spite of that fact, they are worth attention beyond that justified by their frequency because of light they may bring to bear upon the subject of pancreatic neoplasia in general.

This paper presents a case of pancreatic carcinoma in a child, reviews the literature on the subject of tumors of nonendocrine pancreatic epithelium in children, and offers a system of classification based upon presumed histogenesis of carcinoma of the pancreas in young individuals.

Tumors related to the gut–endocrine system ('islet-cell' adenomas, 'islet-cell' adenocarcinomas, etc.) will receive no further consideration in this discussion beyond the statement that even this tidy dissociation breaks down increasingly as the sophistication by which lesions are studied increases the recognition of mixed endocrine and nonendocrine types [1].

1. REPORT OF A CASE

L.S., a 6-year old white girl, was admitted to St. Louis Children's Hospital with a palpable left upper abdominal mass. Upper abdominal radiographic studies showed a focally calcified left upper quadrant mass displacing the stomach anteriorly and superiorly. Urinalysis, hemogram, and intravenous pyelogram were normal. At laparotomy on November 13, 1968, the liver was found to be studded with $2 \times 1 \times 1.5$ cm white nodules. A large mass, deemed unresectable, was obvious in the left upper quadrant extending from the retroperitoneal space into the transverse mesocolon. A hepatic nodule was biopsied. The pathologic diagnosis was neuroblastoma. A sample of tumor tissue placed in tissue culture grew with a pattern suggesting

G. B. Humphrey et al. (eds.), Pancreatic Tumors in Children.
© *1982 Martinus Nijhoff Publishers, The Hague/Boston/London.* ISBN-13:978-94-009-7617-7

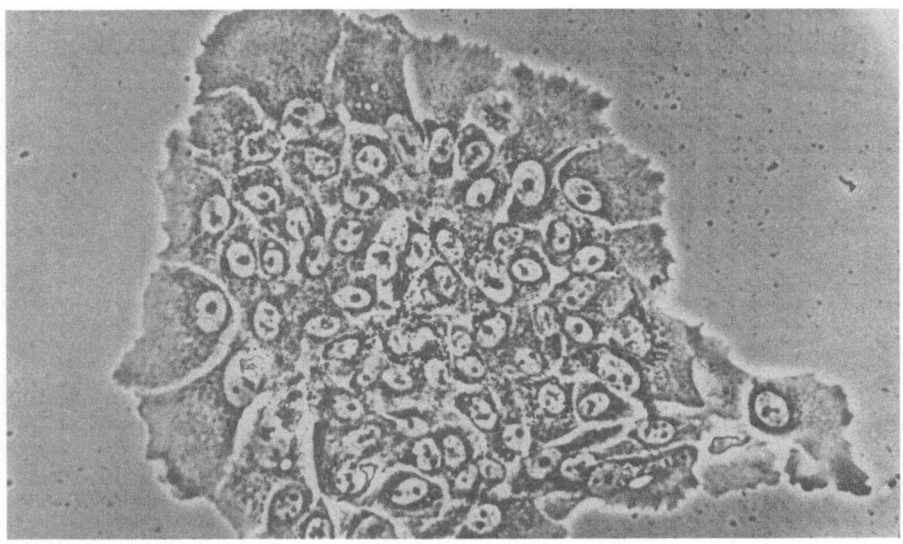

Figure 1. Case #32. Photomicrograph of tumor from biopsy grown in a tissue culture. The cohesive, pavement-like array is typical of epithelial cells (dark field illumination, ×

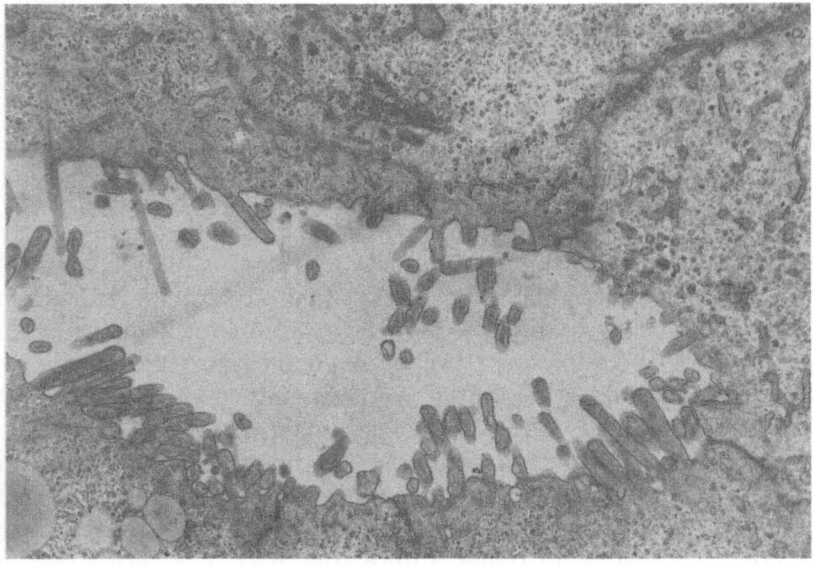

Figure 2. Case #32. Electron micrograph of tumor tissue from second operation. Portions of six cells are seen surrounding a lumen. The luminal surface bears microvilli and there are membrane junctions between cells. These features are typical of differentiation to ducts.

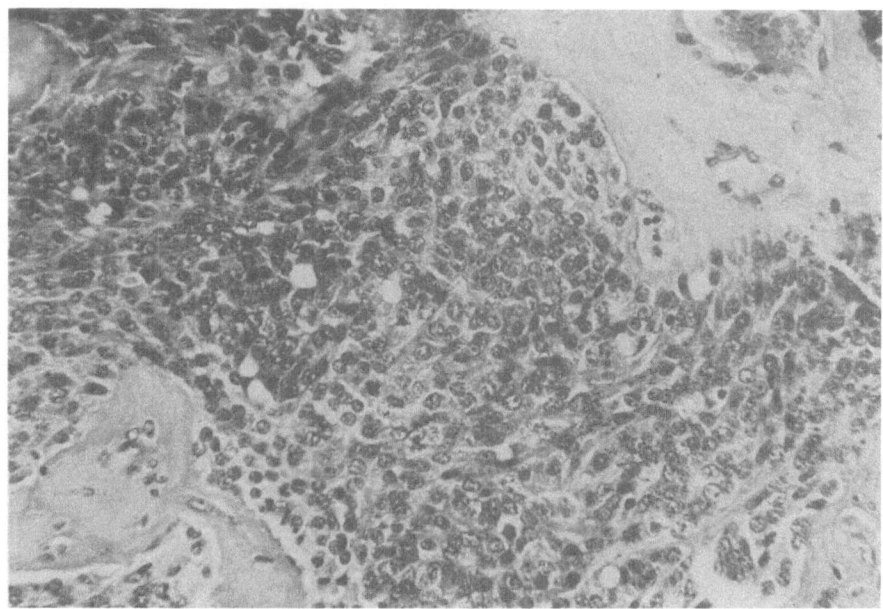

Figure 3. Case #32. Pancreatoblastoma, solid and papillary type; photomicrograph showing a solid area of tumor cells between fibrous trabeculae (H & E, × 245).

epithelial origin unlike the pattern of growth of a neuroblastoma (Figure 1).* The patient received radiation therapy and chemotherapy, cytoxan and vincristine. The abdominal mass slowly increased in size until, 13 months later, the patient developed intractible diarrhea. A peroral jejunal biopsy was normal. On December 3, 1970, a segmental resection of the transverse colon was performed along with splenectomy and removal of a retroperitoneal mass involving the tail of the pancreas. The pathologic diagnosis remained neuroblastoma. Cultured tumor tissue grew in a ductal pattern with microvilli and membrane specializations (Figure 2).

The patient returned to the hospital sixteen months later with a polypoid 5.5 cm recurrence in the colonic suture line which was resected on March 24, 1972. She died at home on April 23, 1972.** Autopsy was not performed.

* Tissue culture studies were performed and illustrations contributed by Milton Goldstein, Ph.D., Department of Anatomy, Washington University School of Medicine.
** I am grateful to Lawrence W. O'Neal, M.D. for follow-up information.

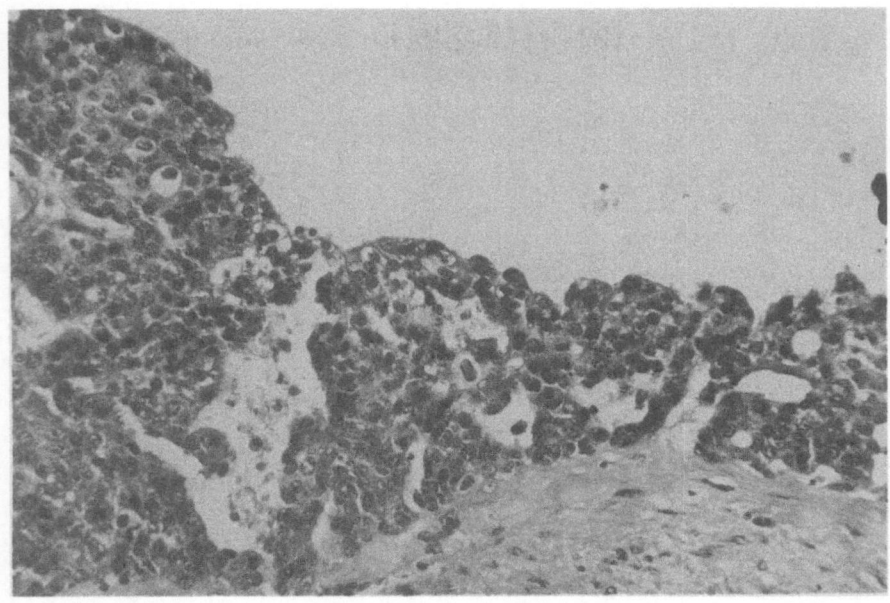

Figure 4. Case #32. Photomicrograph of cribroform papillary area resting on a fibrous septum (H & E, ×245).

1.1. Pathologic Examination

The gross specimen from the second procedure consisted of a nodular, irregular, hemorrhagic mass measuring $8.5 \times 7 \times 3.5$ cm, a 66-gm normal spleen, and 10 cm of attached colon. On section the mass consisted of grey-white nodules of tumor tissue and areas of grumous material. The mass was continuous with the tail of the pancreas.

Microscopically tumor tissue from all three procedures was similar. The tumor was quite pleomorphic. The commonest pattern consisted of structureless sheets of polygonal cells of moderate size with indefinite cell borders, central round or oval nuclei with coursely-stippled chromatin and often a single nucleolus (Figure 3). Among cells with predominantly clear cytoplasm was a random admixture of presumably effete cells with smaller, more chromatic nuclei and more eosinophilic cytoplasm. Fine calcification occupied broad fields of necrosis in the tumor. Occasionally, the tumor tissue which lined some of the spaces seen grossly assumed an arcade-like interanastomosing papillary pattern (Figure 4).

The tumor was traversed by dense trabecula of poorly-cellular fibrous connective tissue continuous with a dense capsule which was, however, infiltrated by nests and strands of tumor cells. The contiguous pancreatic

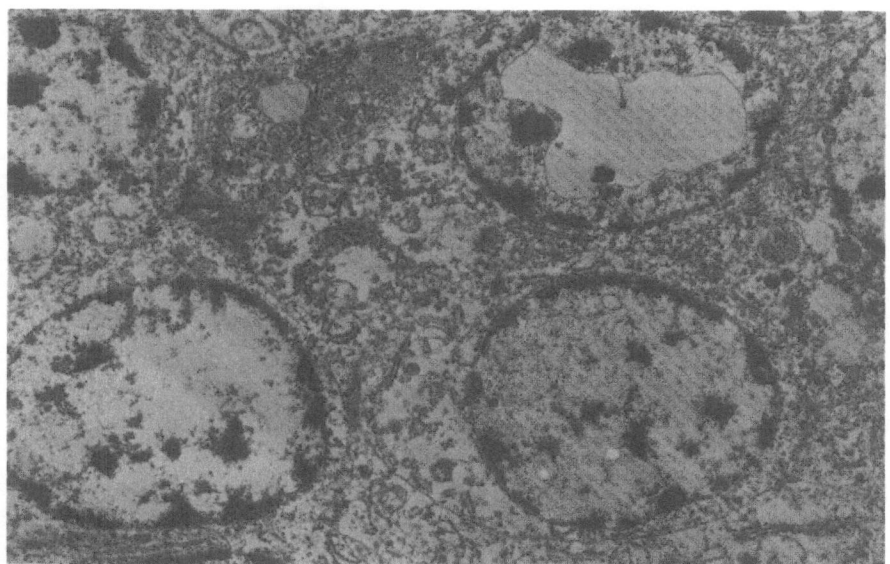

Figure 5. Case # 32. Electron micrograph of formalin-fixed tumor tissue. Tumor cells lack specific secretory granules.

tissue was compressed but normal. Aldehyde fuchsin, phosphotungstic acid hematoxylin, Grimelius and Fontana-Masson stains were negative in the tumor tissue.

Electron microscopy of tumor tissue removed at the third surgical procedure showed solid sheets of polyhedral cells with membrane junctions, limited numbers of organelles, and some glycogen granules. No cytoplasmic secretory granules were identified (Figure 5). Pathologic diagnosis in retrospect is pancreatoblastoma, solid and papillary type (see Discussion).

2. DISCUSSION

Both developmental and acquired cystic lesions occur in the pancreas in infancy and childhood [2, 3, 4]. These very rare nonneoplastic lesions will not be discussed further here beyond calling attention to their consideration in the clinical and morphologic differential diagnosis of tumefactions which arise in the pancreas. It should be noted that cystic fibrosis, in spite of its name, almost never gives rise to clinically or morphologically significant cysts of the pancreas.

2.1. Benign Tumors of Nonendocrine Pancreatic Epithelium

In curious and paradoxical contrast with the salivary glands, the exocrine pancreas rarely gives rise to benign tumors. This principal, true at any age, becomes a virtual interdiction in the case of the infantile or juvenile pancreas. There are almost literally no recorded examples of true adenomas of the exocrine pancreas in infancy or childhood.

2.1.1. Dermoid Cyst.
De Courcy described a 5-cm dermoid cyst of the pancreas in a 2-year old girl and cited two prior examples, both in adults [5].

2.1.2. Adenomas.
Frantz described acinar adenomas as 'the rarest of all benign adenomas if such exists.' [6]. Webb described as an acinar adenoma a 1-mm encapsulated nodule found incidentally at autopsy in the body of the pancreas of a 49-year old man [7]. In evaluating such incidental lesions, one should keep in mind the occurrence of atypical acinar nodules in the pancreas, particularly in individuals with pancreatic carcinoma or a statistically increased risk of developing carcinoma [8]. This is, of course, not ordinarily a consideration in young individuals. I know of no histologic description of an adenoma of the exocrine pancreas in a child.

2.1.3. Cystadenoma.
An uncommon but well-recognized lesion of the pancreas is designated cystadenoma or mucinous cystadenoma. Examples of this tumor are more common in the body or tail than in the head of the pancreas, exhibit a definite female preponderance, and occur in middle-aged or elderly individuals. They are bulky circumscribed lesions with somewhat radially-arranged trabeculae of tissue containing and bordering upon varying-sized cysts. They usually possess a central stellate retracted area of scarring.

Microscopically, two variants are distinguishable [9]. A microcystic or spongiform-type features cuboidal cells devoid of mucin production and with clear cytoplasm which line varying sized round cystic spaces in a single row. The clear cytoplasm is a consequence of prominent accumulations of glycogen. This type is described by Compagno and Oertel [10] as microcystic adenoma (glycogen-rich cystadenoma). These authors studied 34 cases, none from a patient younger than 30 years of age, and this was invariably a benign lesion.

The other variant is designated macrocystic type by Bogomoletz *et al.* [9]. It features tall columnar, conspicuously mucin-secreting epithelium often thrown into redundant intracystic papillary folds. Recognition of transition to cystadenocarcinoma may be difficult. Indeed Compagno and Oertel insist that no example of this lesion can be dismissed as benign and that recurrence or metastases can occur many years after recognition of the initial lesion.

In any event, members of the cystadenoma–cystadenocarcinoma complex are extraordinarily rare in children. Gruber states that he knows of two reports in children, but the cited authors do not appear in his references [11]. Compagno and Oertel found no patient younger than 20 years among 41 examples in the files of the Armed Forces Institute of Pathology [12]. Large collections in the literature fail to include cases in childhood [13–16].

Gille and co-workers described and illustrated a 'cystadenoma' of the pancreas in an infant of 2 years [17]. Judging from the nice photographs, this was a macrocystic variant of the cystadenoma–cystadenocarcinoma complex. The patient survived excision to leave the hospital healthy. The case of Gundersen and Janis in a 16-months old boy was styled as cystadenoma [18]. Actually there were two pancreatic cysts, one large and multi-locular, and several cysts in the transverse mesocolon. This sounds like an example of some developmental cystic lesion, difficult to classify from available information, but not a cystadenoma.

Case #1 in the communication of Grosveld et al. was resected from an 18-month old girl [19]. The lesion was diagnosed pathologically as a benign cystadenoma and is not described further or illustrated. Curiously, the tumor recurred, metastasized, and led to the death of this patient 13 months after the first operation. Metastases had the appearance of a rhabdomyosarcoma, an evolution unique in the authors experience and in mine. One thinks of reported examples of supervention of rhabdomyosarcoma in cases of cystic adenomatoid formation of the lung [20].

The case reported by Mozes and Bogokowsky as a papillary cystadenocarcinoma of the pancreas in a fifteen-year old girl is obviously a pancreatoblastoma of the solid and papillary type [21].

A case record from Massachusetts General Hospital involved a 'papillary adenocystoma' of the pancreas of a 17-year old girl [22]. The lesion is neither illustrated nor described, but the youth of the patient, her sex, and the obvious tendency of the lesion to bleed (her red blood count was 2,500,000 per cumm) suggest that this too may have been an example of a solid and papillary pancreatoblastoma.

2.2. Malignant Tumors

Carcinoma of the pancreas, the fourth commonest cause of death from cancer in the United States, is extraordinarily rare in infants or children. Current thinking regards carcinoma of the pancreas as an environmentally-mediated disease, a supposition with which the rarity of the lesion in young individuals would be in accord. The first cases with histological examination appear to have been Bohn's in 1885, Kuhn's in 1887 followed by Simon's in 1889 and Kaufmann's in 1922 [23–26]. These cases antedate current nomenclature of pancreatic neoplasms, to say nothing of preceding identification of gut–endocrine derived ('islet-cell') tumors. They are, moreover, not illustrated. Admitting the fallibility of interpretation of pathologic designations without illustrations or even much in the way of descriptions, there seems no reason to doubt that each of these lesions was a carcinoma. References to even earlier lesions, perhaps apocryphal [27] and in any event, lacking microscopic examination, are available [11, 28, 29]: the report of Stewart and Stewart is of an autopsy limited to a surgical incision [30]. The pathologic diagnosis of medullary cancer is insuffucient to establish that the lesion was primary in the pancreas. The description by Kochina and Jakovlev [31] of a case reported as a pancreatic cancer with hepatic metastases in a 2-year, 10-month old boy whose sister had died of a malignant renal tumor contains no pathologic details.

Frantz in 1957 counted 14 examples in children of pancreatic carcinoma examined microscopically [6]. In reporting a case in 1976, Taxy tabulated 16 cases from the literature in English [32]. Kakudo and co-workers studied a case in Japan [33]. Horie and co-workers added two cases in 1977 and Benjamin and Wright related two more in 1980 [34, 35]. Without claiming literal completeness, I know of a few other examples [36–38].

2.2.1. Sex. Carcinoma of the pancreas in adults is twice as common in males as in females. In children, although the numbers are inconsequential, the sex distribution of carcinoma is approximately equal. The lesion described by Compagno and Oertel as a 'solid and papillary epithelial neoplasm', however, appears predominantly in young women (see below) [39].

2.2.2. Age. Benjamin and Wright have tabulated the age incidence of pancreatic carcinoma in children and call attention to a bimodal distribution, a peak at 4 years and another at 17 years of age [35]. Again, numbers are small.

2.2.3. Race. Tsukimoto, reporting a case in 1973, collected twelve cases from reports in Japanese literature [40]. This observation raised potentially provocative possibilities of an ethnic 'pocket' in the incidence of pancreatic carcinoma in childhood. I have not been able to verify several citations in this report as transliterated. Among cases accessible to me, four were Japanese [33, 34, 39], one was black ([19], Case #3) and one Chinese [41].

2.2.4. Signs and Symptoms. The presence of a detectable epigastric mass is the commonest clinical feature of pancreatic carcinoma in children [42]. Jaundice, pain and weight loss are less common, in contrast with the prominence of these manifestations in adults.

2.2.5. Diagnosis. Pancreatic carcinoma enters the differential diagnosis of upper abdominal retroperitoneal masses. Interstitial calcification has been seen radiographically ([19], Case #3, [34, 21, 2, 1], and this report) and morphologically and may suggest the much more likely diagnosis of neuroblastoma ([40, 43], and this report). That diagnosis has been made morphologically as well as radiographically in cases of pancreatic carcinoma in childhood. Clinical and laboratory aspects of pancreatic function, either exocrine or endocrine, have been normal. One patient had glycosuria [44]. Humoral agents which would suggest an islet-cell neoplasm have not been detected. In Nanson's case, a duodenal ulcer was present but it was continuous with the centrally necrotic tumor mass in the head of the pancreas [45].

Table 1. Pancreatic epithelial tumors

---

epithelial tumors of nonendocrine origin
  Benign tumors
    Adenomas
      Clear cell adenoma
      Acinar cell adenoma
    Dermoid cyst
  Malignant tumors
    Duct (ductular) cell origin
      Duct cell adenocarcinoma
      Giant cell carcinoma
      Giant cell carcinoma (epulis with osteoid)
      Adenosquamous carcinoma
      Microadenocarcinoma
      Mucinous ('colloid') carcinoma
      Cystadenocarcinoma
    Acinar cell origin
      Acinar cell adenocarcinoma
    Tumors of the immature pancreas, pancreatoblastomas
      Pleomorphic type, acinar differentiation
      Solid and papillary type, ductal or ductular differentiation
    Mixed type: acinar, duct, and islet-cell carcinoma
    Unclassified
      Large cell
      Small cell
      Clear cell
Epithelial tumors of the gut–endocrine system ('islet-cell tumors' etc., benign and malignant) not described in this paper

---

2.2.6. Classification. No system of classification of carcinoma of the pancreas currently enjoys the virtually unanimous acceptance afforded to nomenclatures of certain other organ systems. The systematization of carcinoma of the nonendocrine pancreas recently promulgated by Cubilla and Fitzgerald is morphologically precise and relatively unambiguous [46]. For the present, at least, it can legitimately be made the cornerstone of a system of classification which can be modified, and perhaps even persuasively, expanded to include carcinomas of the pancreas in childhood (Table 1).

2.3. Adenocarcinoma

This is the designation I use for carcinoma of the pancreas in young individuals which is essentially indistinguishable from that which occurs in adults—a moderately well-differentiated adenocarcinoma usually with foci of glandular, ductular or tubular differentiation, often with histologically demonstrable mucin production and often conspicuously demonstrable mucin production and often conspicuously desmoplastic. This is the carcinoma of duct (ductular) cell origin of Cubilla and Fitzgerald. Among reported cases in children, 17 have these features (Table 2) [23–26, 28, 36, 37, 40, 44, 45, 47–53]. I have not included cases interpreted as nonfunctioning islet-cell carcinomas [54–56], but lacking electron microscopy, distinction of islet-cell neoplasms from nonendocrine pancreatic carcinoma may be difficult.

Grossly, adenocarcinomas ranged from 1.5 to 10 cm in diameter. The lesion described by Simon was 'two-fist size' [25]. Two were simply 'large' [44, 52], and the tumor in Smith's case completely replaced the pancreas [48]. In Nanson's case, a 5-cm spherical mass in the head of the pancreas communicated with a duodenal ulcer and consisted of a centrally excavated mass with a nodular solid rim [45]. Only three tumors failed to involve the head of the pancreas [26, 50, 53].

Microscopically, these lesions have been variously described. From descriptions and available illustrations, the stereotype emerges of a moderately well-differentiated carcinoma with a glandular, ductular or tubular pattern. Only the case of Sanan *et al.* was described as 'poorly differentiated' [52]. The case of Tsukimoto *et al.* contained undifferentiated foci which suggested neuroblastoma [40]. In Corner's case and that of Stout and Todd, desmoplasia drew attention [44, 47]. Morlock and Dockerty described neural invasion [51]. Both of these latter features are often conspicuous in cases of carcinoma of the pancreas in adults. In several cases [28, 47, 48] transitions from normal acinar areas were described, an observation seemingly at odds with the classification of them as tumors of ductal or ductular origin. I suggest that this description not be taken too seriously. At the time in the history of surgical pathology from which these reports emanate, much was

Table 2. Carcinoma of the pancreas in children

No.	Author, year, Reference	Age/sex	Location; gross features	Microscopic features	Speical studies	Follow-up
ADENOCARCINOMA						
1)	Bohn 1885 [23]	7 mo/F	Head; hepatic and lymph node metastases	Adenocarcinoma	None	Died/autopsy
2)	Kuhn 1887 [24]	2 yr/F	Almost replacing pancreas; hepatic and lymph node metastases	Adenocarcinoma	None	Died/autopsy
3)	Simon 1889 [25]	13 yr/M	Two-filt size mass in head; through mucosa of duodenum; hepatic, lymph node, renal metastases	Adenocarcinoma	None	Died/autopsy
4)	Kaufmann 1922 [26]	19 yr/F	Tail; hepatic (3300 gm) and pulmonary lymphatic metastases	'Carcinoma solidum'; no photomicrograph	None	None/presumable died
5)	Stout and Todd 1932 [47]	4 yr/M	2 cm mass in head and body; hepatic and lymph node metastases	Pleomorphic ductal tumor; desmoplasia	None	Died 2 hr post-operation/autopsy
6)	Mielcarek 1935 [28]	15 yr/M	7 cm mass in head obstructing common duct; hepatic and lymph node metastases	Anaplastic cylindrical to spindle cells with acidophilic cytoplasm; transition from acini; vascular invasion	None	Died 5 mo; no surgery/autopsy

Table 2. (Continued)

No.	Author, year, Reference	Age/sex	Location; gross features	Microscopic features	Speical studies	Follow-up
7)	Smith 1935 [48]	14 8/12 yr/M	Complete replacement of pancreas; metastases in liver, lung, adrenals stomach, and lymph nodes	Pleomorphic tumor with alveolar pattern; transition with acini	None	Died 1 mo; no surgery/autopsy
8)	Jeanneney and Laporte 1936 [36]	17 yr/F	Hepatic and lymph node metastases	Trabecular and adenoid carcinoma	None	Diagnostic biopsy/ died/autopsy
9)	Kaletcheff 1939 [37]	14 yr/F	2000 gm tumor; hepatic and lymph node metastases; mammary enlargement	Carcinoma	None	Died 3-week course/autopsy
10)	Comer 1943 [44]	8 mo/F	Large mass in head; hepatic, pleural and lymph node metastases; liver 1680 gm	Very well-differentiated tubular structures, desmoplastic	None	Died 2 hr post-operation/autopsy
11)	Warthen et al. 1952 [49]	15 mo/M	5 cm mass, head and body; metastases in porta hepatis, spleen lung	Embryonal carcinoma; many opinions (see discussion)	None	Died/autopsy
12)	Grant and Percival 1954 [50]	16 yr/F	5 cm mass in body and tail; pulmonary and hepatic metastases	Well-differentiated ducts; no photomicrograph	None	Died 5 mo after symptoms/no surgery/autopsy
13)	Nanson 1954 [45]	17 yr/F	5 cm mass in head; centrally excavated communicating with duodenal ulcer	Glandular, vascularized tumor; little atypia; capsular invasion; transition with acinar areas	None	None

Table 2. (Continued)

No.	Author, year, Reference	Age/sex	Location; gross features	Microscopic features	Speical studies	Follow-up
14)	Morlock and Dockerty 1959 [51]	17 yr/M	6 cm mass in head and body invading portal vein; hepatic metastases	'Grade 2' tumor invading nerves, producing mucin	None	None
15)	Sanan et al. 1968 [52]	17 yr/F	Large mass in head obstructing common duct and small bowel	Poorly-differentiated adenocarcinoma	None	Died 9 wks post-operation/autopsy
16)	Tsukimoto et al. 1973 [40]	4 yr/F	10 cm mass in head; hepatic metastases	Adenocarcinoma with areas of 'carcinoma simplex'; undifferentiated foci suggesting neuroblastoma	None	Died 1 mo post-operation/autopsy
17)	Tavassoli and Lynch 1974 [53]	17 yr/F	1.5 cm mass in tail, localized	Well-differentiated tumor; mucin production, signet-ring cells, vascular invasion	None	Incidental finding at autopsy in patient with leukemia, histoplasmosis
ADENOCARCINOMA (acinar type)						
18)	Taxy 1976 [32]	13 yr/F	6.5 × 5 × 4.5 cm mass in head	Focal 'Islet-cell' pattern, acinar and ductal structures, PAS-positive, diastase-resistant granules	E.M. zymogen granules	Alive 3 mo post-operation

112

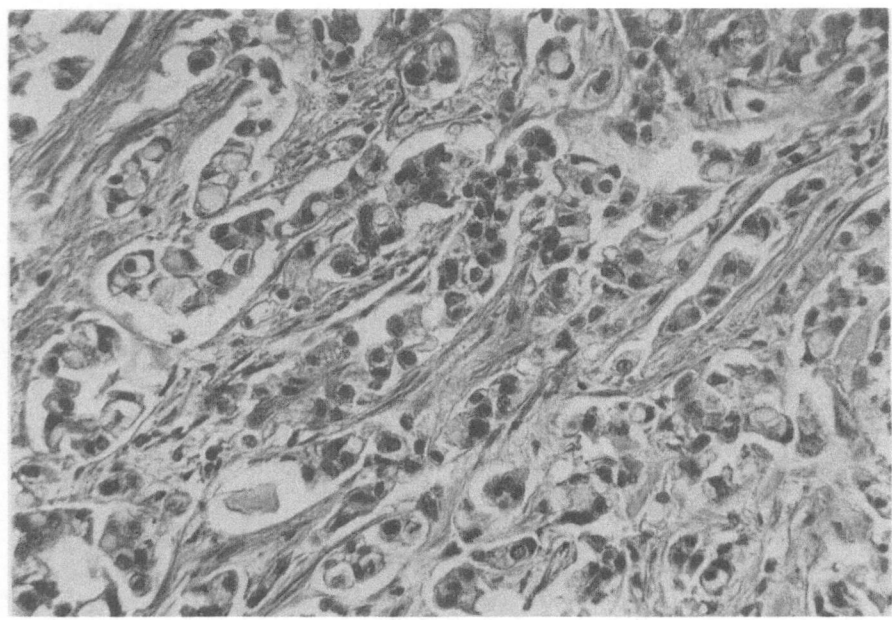

Figure 6. Case #17. Adenocarcinoma of the pancreas in a 17-year old girl. Signet-ring cells are evident (lower left). This figure bears on the case reported by Tavassoli and Lynch [53] H & E, ×245).

made of supposed transitions between normal tissue and the margins of neoplasms. No expert makes much of that phenomenon anymore.

The illustration of Corner's case is very peculiar, depicting a strikingly well-differentiated, bland, tubular lesion [44]. One is tempted to think of the microcystic or clear cell (glycogen-rich) variant of pancreatic cystadenoma (see above) except that that lesion is always benign in the experience of Compagno and Oertel while Corner's case had widespread metastases.

Experience with pancreatic carcinoma in adults makes possible recognition of variously designated histologic variants. Table 1 incorporates Cubilla's and Fitzgerald's systematization, and I have previously made use of a similar one [57]. When one is dealing with a sample of only seventeen cases, it is surely an overrefinement to attempt subclassification even if available descriptions and illustrations were more detailed than they are. In point of fact, further histologic subclassification is not possible. Indeed, such a basic histologic feature as mucin production is specifically mentioned in only two reports [51, 53], and only in the last of these is the description ' signet-ring cells' used. In that lesion, signet-ring cells were not overwhelmingly prominent, and lakes of mucin were absent (Figure 6). Special studies, most spe-

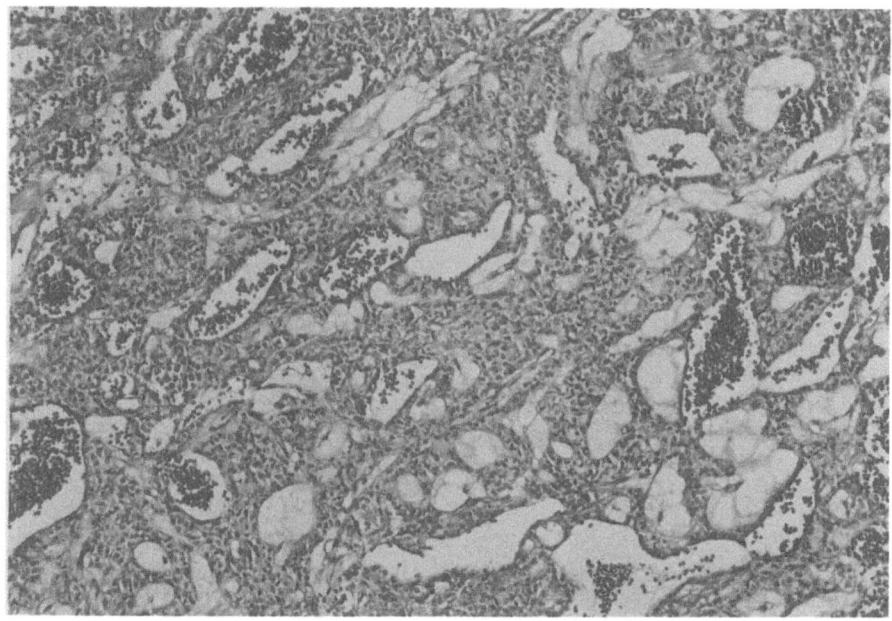

Figure 7. Case #18. Acinar carcinoma; photomicrograph of organoid area interrupted by vascular septa and amphophilic foci rich in acid mucopolysaccharides (H & E, × 105). This figure, together with Figure 8 and 9 pertains to the case reported by Taxy [32]. Material kindly made available by Dr. J.B. Taxy, Johns Hopkins University Medical School, Baltimore, Maryland.

cifically electron microscopic examinations, were applied to no lesion in this group.

In seven cases, surgical procedures varied from biopsy only to attempts at extirpation [36, 40, 44, 47, 50, 51, 52]. Five of these patients died; 2 hrs to 9 weeks after surgery [36, 40, 48, 50, 52]. In Tavassoli and Lynch's case, the carcinoma was an incidental finding at autopsy in a 17-year old girl with leukemia who died of histoplasmosis, a complication of chemotherapy [53]. In two cases no follow-up information is given [45, 51]. No child is known to have survived the diagnosis of pancreatic adenocarcinoma of this type.

2.4. Acinar Carcinoma

In the case reported by Taxy, a 13-year old girl, a right upper quadrant mass had been noted by the patient's mother for two months [32]. The girl indicated that she had been aware of the mass for approximately two years but had ignored it. After biopsy of a mass in the head of the pancreas, pancreatoduonectomy, partial gastrectomy with cholecystectomy was performed, removing a 6.5 × 5 × 4.5 cm pancreatic mass. A thick fibrous capsule separated the mass from the contiguous pancreas. Grossly the tumor

114

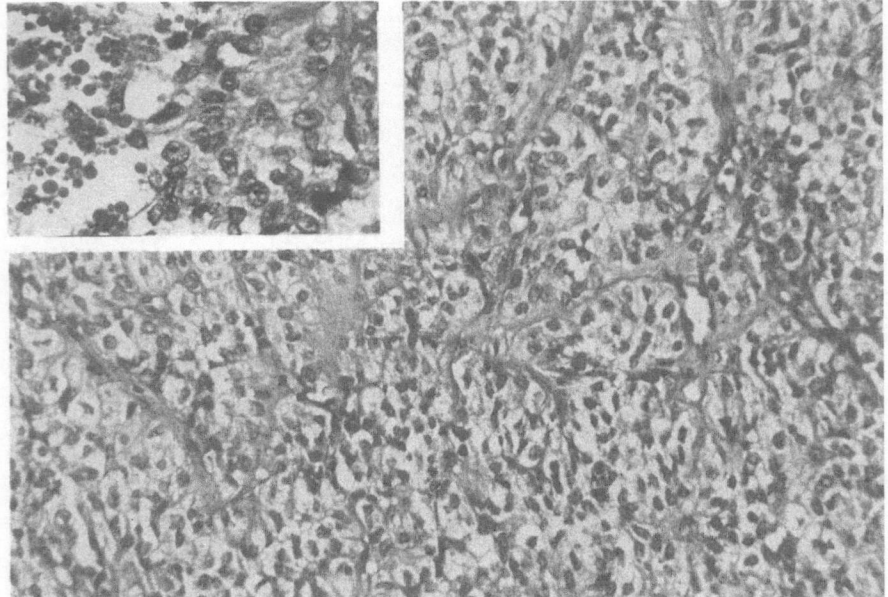

Figure 8. Case #18. Acinar carcinoma; photomicrograph showing ill-defined aggregates of radially arranged cells resting on delicate fibrous septae (H & E, ×245). The inset shows variably-sized round granules in the cytoplasm of neoplastic acinar cells and loose in the interstitium (Masson trichrome, ×420).

was lobulated with a light-brown surface and areas of hemorrhage and degeneration.

Microscopically, the tumor was extensively vascularized. Two patterns were displayed. In some areas, particularly towards the center of the tumor, nests and cords of tumor cells with small dark uniform nuclei and a variable amount of clear cytoplasm were supported by an acellular fibrillar amphophilic stroma which contained abundant acid mucopolysaccharides (Figure 7). Particularly near the periphery, the tumor was more organoid, suggesting to the author an islet-cell tumor (Figure 8). Here, the cells were plump with uniform, vesicular, regularly chromatic nuclei and stringy eosinophilic cytoplasm. PAS-positive, diastase-resistant granules, particularly in apical region of cells and being released into lumina supported an acinar origin for this neoplasm.

By electron microscopy two types of cells were demonstrated, dark and light, with transitional types. The dark cells had abundant mitochondria, free ribosomes, active Golgi apparatuses and stacks of annulate lamellae. Lysosomes were present in some cells, and a few cells contained zymogen

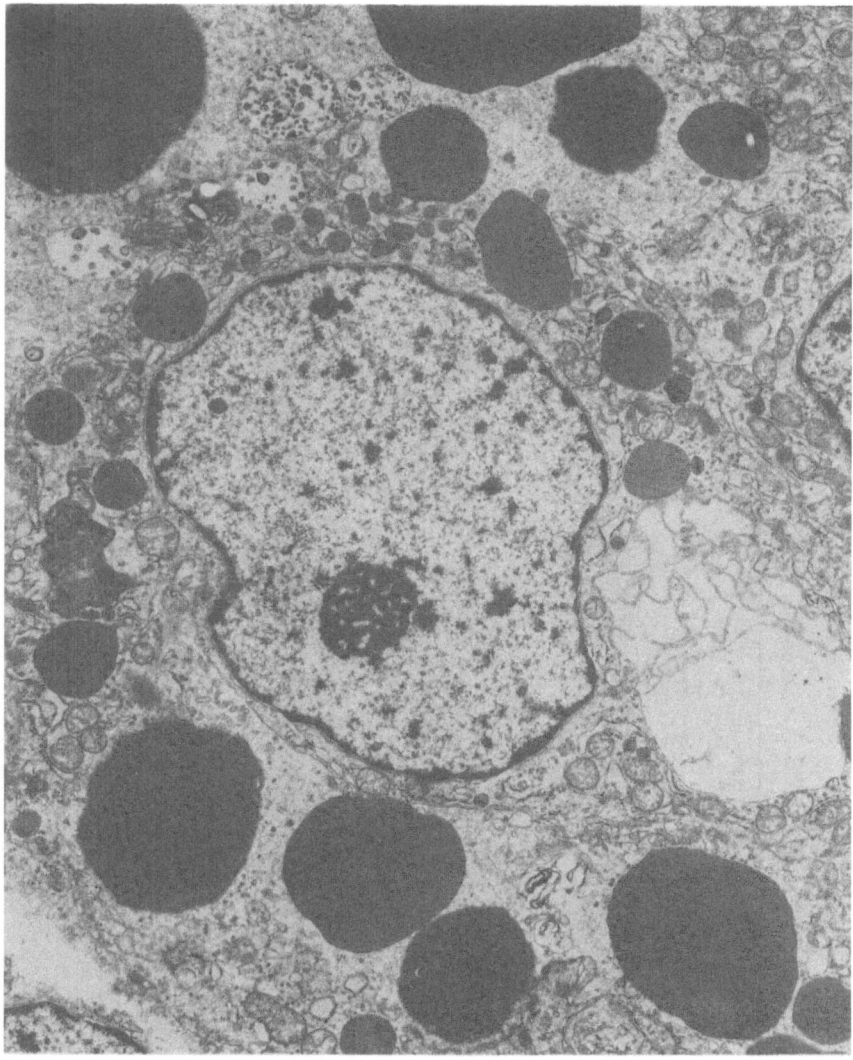

Figure 9. Case #18. Electron micrograph showing a tumor cell which contains many large membrane- bound, electron-dense granules typical of zymogen granules. Print contributed by J.B. Taxy, M.D..

granules (Figure 9). Some of the zymogen granules had rounded pleomorphic central inclusions interpreted as manifestations of degeneration.

Taxy authoritatively reviewed cases reported in English and distinguished twelve cases of nonacinar origin from cases of acinar origin (four including his own). He related his case to others previously reported [19, 43, 58] in

Table 3. Pancreatoblastoma

PLEOMORPHIC TYPE

Author, year, No. reference	Age/sex	Location; gross features	Microscopic features	Special studies	Follow-up
19) Moynan et al. 1964 [43]	5½ yr/F	2.5 cm mass in head; hepatic, renal (left), and lymph node metastases	Spindle and epithelial cells, ductal pattern; mucin in glands; transition with acinar areas	None	Died 9 days post-operation
20) Grosfeld et al. 1970 [19] Case #3	10 yr/M	10 × 12 cm mass in tail; hepatic and peritoneal metastases	Adenocarcinoma of acinar origin	E.M. zymogen precursors	Alive 9 mo post-operation/chemotherapy
21) Frable et al. 1971 [58]	4 yr/F	Large mass in head extending into superior mesenteric vein; transverse colon, and mesentery	Acinar and glandular structures, squamous foci; focal pattern suggesting islet cells. PAS-positive diastase-senstive granules	E.M. zymogen granules	Died 12 days post-operation/autopsy
22) Rosenberg 1973 [38] Case #6	4 yr/F	Pancreas plus mass 180 gm middle third of pancreas	Fibrous capsule, mixture of glandular elements and spindle cells; focal papillae on fibrovascular stalks; PAS-positive secretion in lumina	E.M. both zymogen granules and ductile (sic) elements	Doing well 15 mo
23) Mah et al. 1974 [41]	9 yr/M	9 cm mass in head	Acinar pattern, no ducts; granules positive with dimethylaminobenzaldehyde nitrate stain for tryptophan	None	Died 10 mo post-operation/no autopsy

Table 3. (Continued)

Author, year, No. reference	Age/sex	Location; gross features	Microscopic features	Special studies	Follow-up
24) Kakudo *et al.* 1976 [33]	3 yr/F	249 gram 15 × 5 × 5 cm encapsulated partly cystic mass in tail	Tubulo-acinar tumor, stellate stroma; 'islet-cell carcinoma with vacular invasion'; aldehyde fuchsin and aldehyde thionin stains negative	E.M. two types of cells, one epithelial with microvilli and dark granules and glycogen, the other more primative no microvilli, few organelles, no granules or glycogen	Resected; hepatic metastases, 1 yr later; chemotherapy; abdominal mass 3 yrs later, reexplored, block excision; no metastases in liver
25) Horie *et al.* 1977 [34] Case #1	4 11/12 yr/M	11 × 9 × 8.5 cm encapsulated mass attached to head by fibrovascular stalk	Organoid structures with 3 layers, central squamoid corpuscles, intermediate zone of light cell masses, peripheral tubular structures	None	Alive and well 16 yrs later
26) Case #2	5 11/12 yr/M	Encapsulated mass 7 × 6 × 5 cm adherent to duodenal bulb, mesocolon, and pancreas	Lobular pattern, three layers as in case 1; PAS-positive granules in apical cytoplasm of some cells	E.M. zymogen granules; microvilli	Alive and healthy more than 2 yrs later
27) Benjamin and Wright 1980 [35] Case #1	7 yr/M	11 cm rounded mass in head; central cavity with peripheral nodules	Triphasic PAS-positive, diastase-resistant material: no granules; small islands of squamous epithelium; cartilage in stroma	E.M. granules 300 to 500 nm, tonofilaments; immunoperoidase showed α-1-antitrypsin	Well, 10 mo later
28) Case #2	16 yr/F	Cysti mass, 11 cm diameter, in tail; nodular deposits in greater omentum	Polygonal cells in sheets and small cysts; PAS-positive diastase-resistant granules	E.M. zymogen granules; immunoperoxidase showed α-1-antitrypsin	Well, 2 mo radio-therapy

Table 3. (Continued)

Author, year, No. reference	Age/sex	Location; gross features	Microscopic features	Special studies	Follow-up
SOLID AND PAPILLARY TYPE					
29) Frantz 1959 [6]	2 yr/M	335 gm body and tail	Papillary carcinoma	None	Died post-operation
30) Mozes and Bogokowsky 1963 [21]	15 yr/F	Encapsulated orangesize mass in tail; calcified on X-ray	Palpillary cystadenocarcimona	None	Surgically excised; left hospital
31) Hamoudi *et al.* 1970 [61]	12 yr/F	10 cm encapsulated mass in head	Papillary pattern with focal ribbons	E.M. and histo-chemistry negative for specific granules	Alive 1 yr post-operation/well 1/81
32) Present report 1981	6 yr/F	Large mass in left epigastrium involving tail of pancreas; calcification on X-ray; hepatic metastases	Solid and papillary tumor; interstitial calcifications	Epithelial growth in tissue culture (see text, Figures 3 and 4); ductules by E.M.	Hepatic metastases interpreted as neuroblastoma; chemotherapy, irradiation; resection $8.5 \times 7 \times 3.5$ cm mass involving pancreas 2 yrs later; resection coloni recurrence $2^3/12$ yrs later; died 1 mo post-operation; total course $4^6/12$ yrs

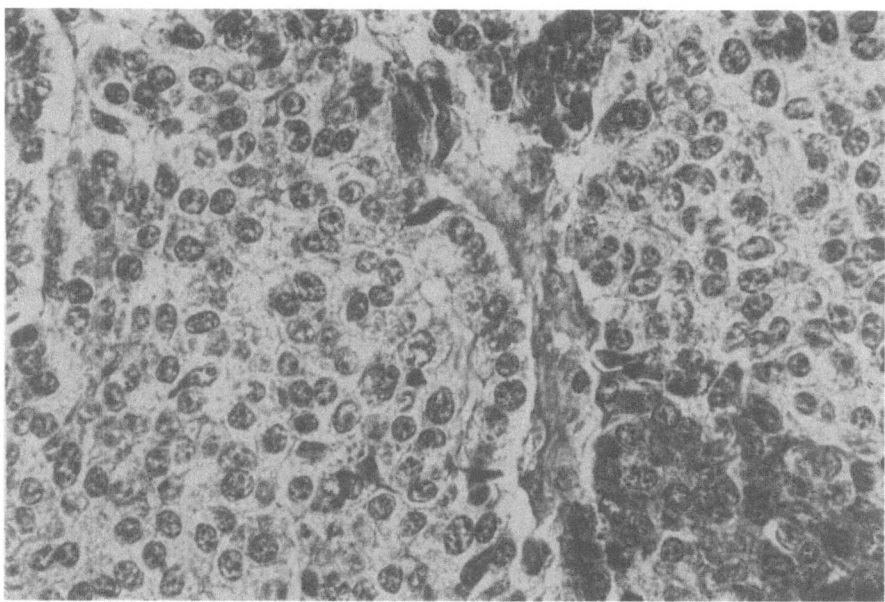

Figure 10. Case #21. Pancreatoblastoma, pleomorphic type; photomicrograph of solid area of tumor cells with transition to a row of cuboidal cells along a fibrous trabecula (H & E, ×630). This figure, together with Figures 11 and 12 pertains to the case reported by Frable *et al.* [58]. Material graciously made available by Dr. W.J. Frable, Medical College of Virginia, Richmond, Virginia.

which zymogen granules had been demonstrated electron microscopically or histochemically [41]. In spite of that, I think Taxy's case is an acinar carcinoma analogous to that which occurs in adults and unrelated to the embryogenesis of the pancreas. When the designation 'acinar carcinoma' is limited to lesions with demonstrable zymogen granules or to cases in which enzymatic activity is demonstrated in tumor tissue or metastases [59], that lesion is very rare even in adults, contributing about one percent of all cases of pancreatic carcinoma [46]. Taxy's case is, in my opinion, the only such lesion reported in a child.

2.5. *Pancreatoblastoma, pleomorphic type*

A distinctive tumor of the pancreas of young individuals has come to be known as 'pancreatoblastoma'. Salient features of 10 reported cases are summarized in Table 3 [19, 33–35, 38, 41, 43, 58]. Patients have ranged from 3 to 16 years of age. Five have been girls, five boys.

Grossly, these have been bulky, bossellated lesions as large as 11 cm in diameter. Several have been encapsulated. The cut surface has been lobular,

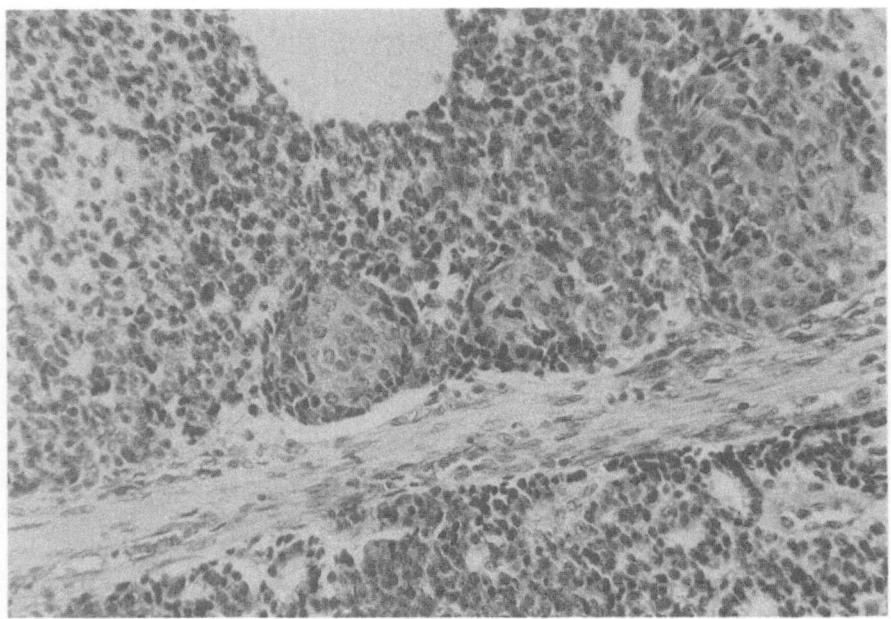

Figure 11. Case #21. Pancreatoblastoma, pleomorphic type. Nests of squamous cells are present in a solid area of tumor cells (H & E, ×245).

grey-white to yellow-white in color and has often manifestated degenerative phenomena, hemorrhage, necrosis and 'cyst formation'.

Microscopically, these lesions are pleomorphic, consisting of two or three patterns. Most basic are structureless sheets of cells of moderate size with indistinct cell borders, clear to finely granular to eosinophilic cytoplasm and a central ovoid nucleus with coursely-stippled chromatin and usually a single nucleolus (Figure 10). In some areas, this pattern merges with fields of alveolar, ductular, or tubular forms lined by the same cells often arranged in an organoid pattern. Very conspicuous in many cases have been round or oval foci of squamous cells (Figure 11) which merge peripherally with fields of pavement-like or spindle-shaped cells, then, still more peripherally, into the structureless areas described above. Mitoses are infrequent. Case #1 of Benjamin and Wright had cartilage in the stroma [35]. Amyloid is not identified in the stroma.

Trichrome stains may demonstrate zymogen granules in tumor cells. In the case of Mah *et al.*, cytoplasmic granules stained with the dimethylaminobenzaldehyde nitrate reaction for tryptophan as do zymogen granules in nonneoplastic acini [41].

In both of Benjamin and Wright's cases a-1-antitrypsin was demonstrated in granular cytoplasmic deposits [35]. Significance of this is not clear.

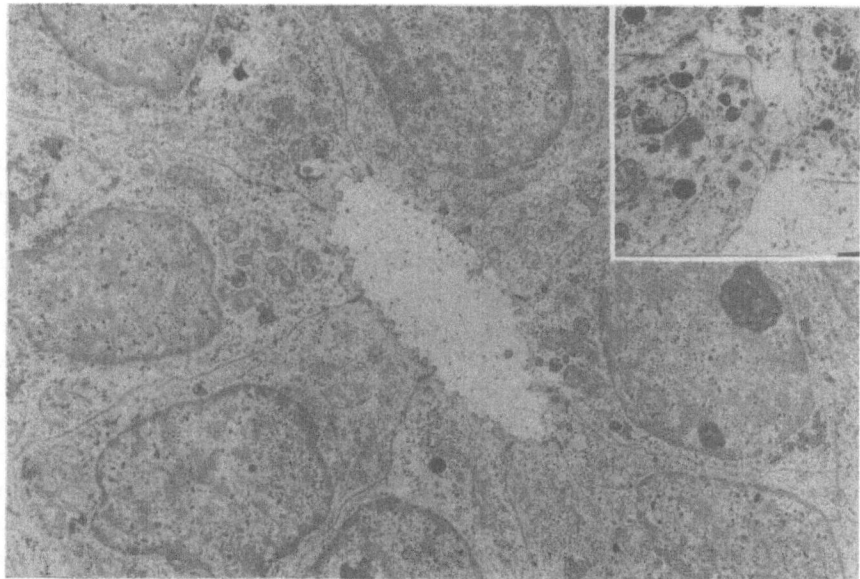

Figure 12. Case #21. Pancreatoblastoma, pleomorphic type; electron micrograph showing ductular structures lined by cells with membrane junctions and microvilli. The pical cytoplasm contains round electron-dense zymogen granules (inset).

Electron microscopy clearly demonstrates an epithelial origin for these tumor cells. There are membrane specializations between contiguous cells, and microvilli protrude into luminal spaces. The cytoplasm usually has a well-developed Golgi complex and stacks of endoplasmic reticulum. Mitochondria are numerous and of moderate size. Most striking is the presence of numerous round, dark electron-dense granules usually 300 to 500 nm in diameter interpreted as zymogen granules or precursors of zymogen granules (Figure 12). Small amounts of glycogen correlate with focal diastase-sensitive cytoplasmic granularity seen light microscopically.

2.5.1. Course. Large size, circumscribed, often frankly encapsulated gross appearance, and scanty mitotic activity are not features of a highly malignant neoplasm. The capsule of these lesions is occasionally described as focally infiltrated, however, and three cases had metastases [33, 34, 42]. One must therefore attribute at least a sluggish malignancy to these lesions. In point of fact, only three of the reported cases are known to have died [41, 43, 58].

2.5.2. Histogenesis. During the histogenesis of the pancreas, acini differentiate from a branching system of tubules which terminate in centroacinar ducts, so called because their lumina are in direct contact with and receive the secretions of the acini. Centroacinar ducts are also capable of giving rise to islets which lose connection with them. A system of tubules also connects small mucous glands of the larger pancreatic ducts with islets, rarely acini. Frable and co-workers associate the histogenesis of the pleomorphic tumor of the pancreas in young individuals (not exclusively infants) to recapitulation of this developmental mechanism [58]. They ascribe these tumors to originate from ductules which have retained the capacity for acinar differentiation. Potency to form squamous cells is also reflected in several reported examples. In one case, tonofilaments and degenerated zymogen granules were observed electron microscopically in the same cells, bespeaking multipotency by the tumor cells [35].

The occurrence of squamous foci in certain carcinomas of the adult pancreas (adenosquamous carcinoma) and even of epidermoid carcinoma is usually related to the tendency of ducts and ductules of the diseased pancreas to undergo squamous metaplasia. I know of no report of adenosquamous carcinoma or epidermoid carcinoma in the pancreas of a child. That the immature pancreas, or derivatives of it, is otherwise capable of squamous differentiation is evinced by the occurrence of squamous foci in a developmental cyst of the pancreas [4] and, of course, in a dermoid cyst [5]. One recalls that squamous foci also occur in some examples of the tumor of the immature liver, hepatoblastoma. Interestingly chrondroid, osteoid and, occasionally true bone can also occur in the stroma of hepatoblastoma. Cartilage was found in the stroma of one reported pancreatoblastoma [35]. The hypothesis that pancreatoblastoma arises from derivatives of the ventral pancreas which does not give rise to islets [34] is not in accord with current evidence regarding embryogenesis of the pancreas.

Squamous foci were specifically described in six cases (Cases #19, 21, 22, 25, 26, 27). The microscopic descriptions of three other cases do not mention squamous foci (Cases #20, 23 and 28). In the case described by Kakudo et al. (Case #24), squamous foci were specifically not seen. The cases tabulated as pleomorphic pancreatoblastoma share the presence of zymogen granules in tumor cells but therefore fall into two subgroups, one with squamous foci in the tumor tissue, the other without. Whether this is a true biologic difference or the result of variable sampling is not clear.

2.6. Pancreatoblastoma, Solid and Papillary Type

On page 33 of her 1959 fascicle on tumors of the pancreas, Frantz illustrated three examples of 'Papillary tumors of the pancreas—benign or malignant?' All three patients were young individuals, a 20-year old woman, a 2-year old boy and a 24-year old woman [6].

Table 3 summarizes four detailed reports of this lesion in the litera-

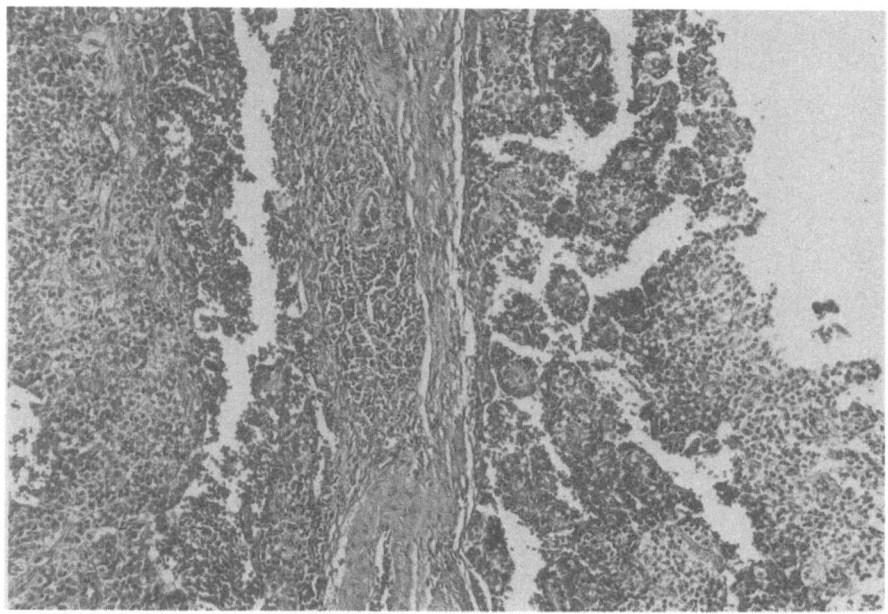

Figure 13. Pancreatoblastoma, solid and papillary type; photomicrograph from an unreported case showing papillary (right) and solid areas (left) (H & E, × 105). Material for this figure and for Figures 14 and 15 were kindly supplied by Dr. John Compagno, Oakland Naval Hospital, Oakland, California.

ture [6, 21, 61], but that figure does not represent its relative frequency. In the first place, we have not included two of Frantz's cases (20- and 24-year old women) nor the case illustrated by Gruber (his p. 510), also a young adult women [11]. Recently, Oertel and co-workers have studied fifty-two examples of this lesion, a 'solid and papillary epithelial neoplasm, probably of small duct origin'. Only an abstract of this experience has been published [39], but salient features include young patients (average age 24 years) bulky lesions, often encapsulated, often hemorrhagic, with a striking predilection to appear in adolescent girls or young women. Cubilla and Fitzgerald have encountered one example of a 'papillary cystic tumor' but give no details [46]. Hamoudi and co-workers characterized the lesion in their case (also Case #2 of Grosfeld) as a 'papillary epithelial neoplasm' and recognized its identity with the lesions illustrated by Frantz [61]. The case presentation in this report also exemplifies this lesion.

Like the pleomorphic pancreatoblastoma, these too are bulky lesions many centimeters in diameter. The illustration (his p. 510) in Gruber's chapter of a lesion found incidentally at autopsy in a young woman who

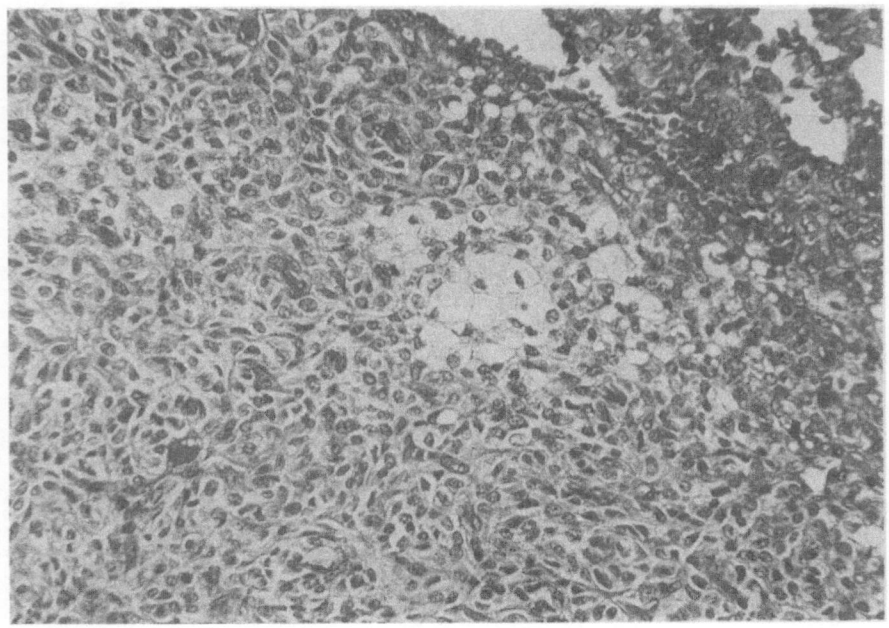

Figure 14. Pancratoblastoma, solid and papillary type; photomicrograph showing foam cells in a solid area of tumor cells (H & E, × 63).

died of tuberculous peritonitis is typical [11]. The cut surface has often been hemorrhagic with pseudocyst formation.

Microscopically solid and papillary fields alternate, often abruptly (Figure 13). The solid areas consist of sheets of polyhedral cells with indistinct cell borders and clear or pale cytoplasm. Nuclei are central, round or oval with stippled chromatin and usually a single nucleolus. Mitotic figures are sparse. A dense, poorly cellular fibrous capsule, sometimes infiltrated by tumor cells, sends fascicles into the interior of the tumor dividing it into ill-defined lobules. These areas merge abruptly into areas of densely-arranged papillary or microtubular forms lined by the same cells as occur in the solid areas but arranged as single or multilayered rows over fibrovascular stalks. A peculiar interstitial formation of foam cells (Figure 14) and even cholesterol granulomata (Figure 15) has been present in two examples I have seen, and correlates with the stippled calcification seen radiographically in the mass in several cases ([6], p. 33, [21], and this report). These foci occur abruptly in solid lobules of fully viable tumor tissue, not, as one might except, in or adjoining areas of necrosis or hemorrhage although such areas are abundant.

Electron microscopy has been interpreted as suggesting a ductal origin for

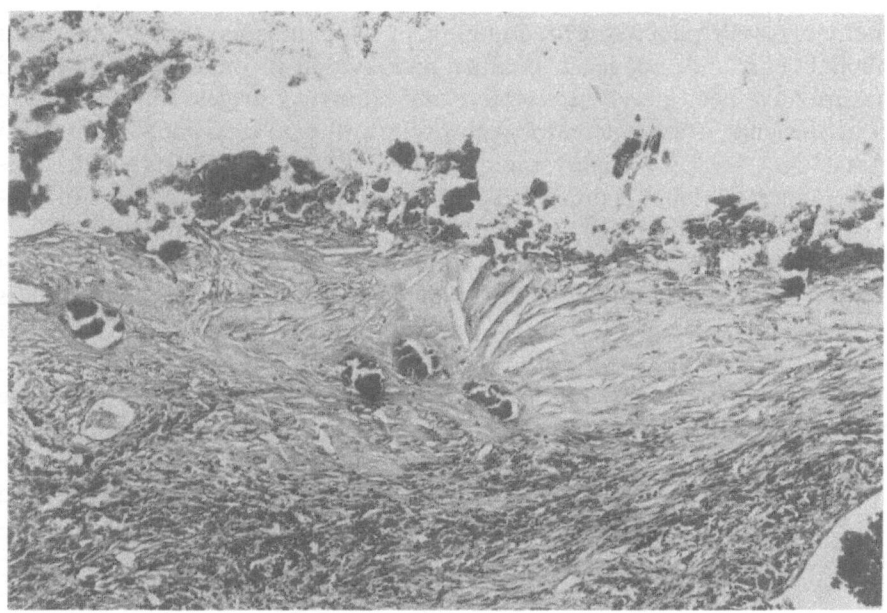

Figure 15. Pancreatoblastoma, soliid and papillary type; photomicrograph showing cholesterol granuloma and an area of calcification (H & E, ×63).

these neoplasms. The tumor cells have membrane intercellular specializations and scanty microvilli protruding into luminal spaces. Mitochondria are of moderate size and abundant. Annulate lamellae and cytoplasmic tonofilaments have been described. No granules have been identified in these lesions.

2.6.1. Course. The course of these tumors is sluggishly malignant with prolonged survival possible even in the presence of proven metastases. Only one of the 52 cases studied by Compagno *et al.* died of distant metastases [39], but our patient had hepatic metastases when she was first seen and died four and a half years later.

2.6.2. Histogenesis. The ductal origin suggested by many authors for these tumors would seem to be amply confirmed by the tissue culture studies of tumor tissue reported herein. The heterogeneity of the lesion as well as its occurrence in young individuals suggests an origin in the incompletely differentiated pancreas much as pulmonary blastomas, most of which occur in adults, are thought to be related to the embryogenesis of the lung.

Because, like the more strikingly pleomorphic type of pancreatoblastoma, these lesions occur in young individuals and seem to recapitulate the development of small pancreatic ductules from solid masses of less organized epithelial cells, and, not least, because names used in the as yet unfocused literature have been purely descriptive and clumsy, I suggest that this lesion also be designated as pancreatoblastoma but of *solid and papillary* type in contrast with the presumably more primative, *pleomorphic* type. Perhaps the two types of lesion represent development from different stages of precursor cells. Transitional or intermediate types may be anticipated.

The absence of squamous foci in three or four cases (Cases #20, 23, 24 and 28) here tabulated and considered as pleomorphic pancreatoblastoma is difficult to interpret in view of the limited number of cases. Perhaps that absence represents a sampling problem in dealing with a bulky neoplasm. On the other hand it may represent a true biologic difference in that these tumors with acinar differentiation represented by the presence of zymogen granules may fall by other morphologic considerations between the more frequent pleomorphic pancreatoblastoma with squamous foci and the solid and papillary pancreatoblastoma with neither zymogen granules nor squamous foci.

3. SUMMARY

The subject of tumors of the nonendocrine pancreatic epithelium in young individuals is reviewed and supplemented by a case report. Carcinoma of the exocrine pancreas, very rare in children, appears to fall into three phenomenologic groups:
a) A group of cases indistinguishable from carcinoma of the pancreas in adults. All patients reported in detail have died, usually with distant metastases.
b) Pancreatoblastoma, pleomorphic type, a tumor of sluggish malignancy featuring a pleomorphic histological pattern, foci of squamous differentiation and differentiation towards acinar cells.
c) Pancreatoblastoma, solid and papillary type, with a proclivity to involve females, sluggish malignancy and recapitulation in tissue culture of ductule or ductular differentiation.

It is suggested that the last two types may be systematically related and that lesions with features intermediate between the two typical extremes may be anticipated.

ACKNOWLEDGEMENTS

I am grateful to many physicians for their interest and cooperation during preparation of this communication. They gave freely of their time, experience, and opinions and willingly made material available for me to examine. I deeply appreciate their help and at the same time absolve them of responsibility for the interpretations I have drawn. Their number includes: J.E. Oertel, M.D.; John Compagno, M.D.; W.J. Frable, M.D.; Jerome Taxy, M.D.; Ala B. Hamoudi, M.D.; William Newton, M.D.; L.P. Dehner, M.D.; W. Yudt, M.D.; Harvey Rosenberg, M.D. Mrs. Shirley Price searched out material from our case and prepared some of the electron micrographs. Miss Debra Danieley cheerfully typed the manuscript.

REFERENCES

1. Sommers SC, Meissner WA: Unusual carcinomas of the pancreas. Arch Pathol 58:101-111, 1954.
2. DeLange D, Janssen TAE: Large solitary pancreatic cyst and other developmental errors in a premature infant. Am J Dis Cild 75:587-594, 1948.
3. McPherson TC, Heersma HS: Diagnosis and treatment of pancreatic cysts in children with report of a case. J Pediatr 33:213-218, 1948.
4. Miles RM: Pancreatic cyst in the newborn. Case report. Ann Surg 149:576-581, 1959.
5. De Courcy JL: Dermoid cyst of pancreas. Case report. Ann Surg 118:394-395, 1943.
6. Frantz VK: Tumors of the pancreas. In: Atlas of Tumor Pathology, Section Vii. Fasc 27 and 28, Washington, D.C. Armed Forces Institute of Pathology, 1959, pp 1-149.
7. Webb JN: Acinar cell neoplasms of the exocrine pancreas. J Clin Pathol 30:103-112, 1977.
8. Shinozuka M, Lee RE, Dunn JL, Longnecker DS: Multiple atypical acinar cell nodules in the pancreas. Hum Pathol 11:389-391, 1980.
9. Bogomoletz WV, Adnet JJ, Widgren W, Stavrou M, McLaughlin JE: Cystadenoma of the pancreas: a histologic, histochemical and ultrastructural study of seven cases. Histopathology 4:309-320, 1980.
10. Compagno J, Oertel JE: Microcystic adenomas of the pancreas (glycogen-rich cystadenomas). A clinico-pathologic study of 34 cases. Am J Clin Pathol 69:289-298, 1978.
11. Gruber GB: Pathologie der Bauchspeicheldrüse (Mit Ausnahme der Langerhanschen Inseln und Diabetesfrage). In: Handbuch der speziellen pathologischen Anatomie und Histologie, Henke F, Lubarsch D (eds). Berlin, Julius Springer, 1929, pp 211-621.
12. Compagno J, Oertel JE: Mucinous cystic neoplasms of the pancreas with overt and latent malignancy (cystadeno-carcinoma and cystadenoma). A clinico-pathologic study of 41 cases. Am J Clin Pathol 69:573-480, 1978.
13. Becker WF, Welsh RA, Pratt MS: Cystadenoma and cystadenocarcinoma of the pancreas. Ann Surg 161:845-860, 1965.
14. Benson RE, Gordon W: Cystadenoma of the pancreas with presentation of one case and review of twenty-eight cases collected from the medical literature. Surgery 21:353-361, 1947.
15. Glenner GG, Mallory GK: Cystadenoma and related nonfunctional tumors of the pancreas. Pathogenesis, classification and significance. Cancer 9:980-996, 1956.
16. Piper CE Jr, ReMine WH, Priestyle JT: Cystadenomata. Report of 20 cases. JAMA 180: 648-652, 1962.
17. Gille P, Barbier G, LeClerc D, Bauer J: Cystadenome pancréatique chez un enfant de 2 ans. Ann Chir Infantile (Paris) 13:437-442, 1972.

128

18. Gundersen AE, Janis JF: Pancreatic cystadenoma in childhood. Report of a case. J Pediatr Surg 4:478–481, 1969.
19. Grosfeld JL, Clatworthy HW Jr, Hamoudi AB: Pancreatic malignancy in children. Arch Surg 101:370–375, 1970.
20. Ueda K, Gruppo R, Unger F, Martin L, Bove K: Rhabdomyosarcoma of lung arising in congenital cystic adenomatoid malformation. Cancer 40:383–388, 1977.
21. Mozes M, Bogokowsky H: Les cystadenocarcinomes papillaire du pancréas. A propos d'un cas chez une fille de quinze ans. Lyon Chir 59:498–503, 1963.
22. Mallory TB (ed): Case Records of the Massachusetts General Hospital, Case 27262. N Eng J Med 224:1112–1114, 1941.
23. Bohn: Krebs der Leber, der Portalen und des Pankreas bei einem halbjährigen Kinde. Jahr f Kinderh 23:144–146, 1885.
24. Kuhn A: Über primäres Pankreaskarzinom im Kindesalter. Berl Klin Wchnschn 24:494–496, 1887.
25. Simon F: Über ein Pankreaskarzinom bei einem 13 jährigen Knaben. Inaug Diss Greifswald. Abel J, 1889, pp 1–28.
26. Kaufmann E: Lehrbuch der speziellen pathologischen Anatomie für Studierende und Aerzte, Erster Bd. Berlin und Leipzig: Walter de Gruyter, 1922, p 812.
27. Von Sotow: Pankreaskrebs bei jugendlichen. Mittl Kaiserl med Akad z St. Petersburg, 1903.
28. Mielcarek PA: Primary adenocarcinoma of the pancreas in a fifteen-year old boy. Am J Pathol 11:527–533, 1935.
29. Phillip PW: Über Krebsbildungen im Kindesalter. Krebsforsch 5:326–416, 1907.
30. Stewart SC, Stewart LF: A case of cancer of the pancreas in a nine-Year old boy, with notes on other reported cases of cancer in children. Intern Clin 25:118–126, 1915.
31. Kochina T, Jakovlev A: (Malignant Tumors in 2 children in a family) Vop Onkol 8:88–89, 1962 (in Russian).
32. Taxy JB: Adenocarcinoma of the pancreas in childhood. Report of a case and a review of the English language literature. Cancer 37:1508–1518, 1976.
33. Kakudo K, Sakurai M, Miyaji T, Ikeda Y, Satani M, Manabe H: Pancreatic carcinoma in infancy — an electron microscopic study. Acta Pathol Jpn 26:719–726, 1976.
34. Horie A, Yano Y, Kotoo Y, Miwa A: Morphogenesis of pancreatoblastoma, infantile carcinoma of the pancreas. Report of two cases. Cancer 39:247–254, 1977.
35. Benjamin E, Wright DH: Adenocarcinoma of the pancreas of childhood: a report of two cases. Histopathology 4:87–104, 1980.
36. Jeanneney G, Laporte F: Un cas d'épithelioma du pancréas chez une jeune fille de 17 ans. Jour de Med de Bordeaux 113:791–792, 1936.
37. Kaletcheff A: Carcinoma del pancreas en una muchacha de 14 años. Gac med de Caracas 46:394–395, 1939.
38. Rosenberg H: Undifferentiated cell, potentially malignant tumor of the pancreas in a 4-year old child. Cancer Sem 4:245–248, 1973.
39. Compagno J, Oertel JE, Kremzar M: Solid and papillary epithelial neoplasm of the pancreas, probably of small duct origin: a clinico-pathologic study of 52 cases (Abstract) Lab Invest 40:248–249, 1979.
40. Tsukimoto I, Watanabe K, Lin JB, Nakajima T: Pancreatic carcinomas in children in Japan. Cancer 31:1203–1207, 1973.
41. Mah PT, Loo DC, Tock EPC: Pancreatic acinar cell carcinoma in childhood. Am J Dis Child 128:101–104, 1974.
42. Welch KJ: Pancreatic neoplasms. In: Pediatric Surgery, 2nd ed, Mustard WT, Ravitch MW, Snyder WH Jr, Welch KJ, Benson CD (eds). Chicago: Year Book Medical Publishers Inc.,

1969, pp 758-760.

43. Moynan RW, Neerhout RC, Johnson TS: Pancreatic carcinoma in childhood. J Pediatr 65:711-720, 1964.
44. Corner BD: Primary carcinoma of the pancreas in an infant aged seven months. Arch Dis Child 18:106-108, 1943.
45. Nanson EM: An unusual case of carcinoma of the pancreas. Br J Surg 41:439-441, 1954.
46. Cubilla AL, Fitzgerald PJ: Cancer of the pancreas (nonendocrine): a suggested morphologic classification. Semin in Oncol 6:285-297, 1979.
47. Stout BF, Todd DA: Report of a case of primary adenocarcinoma of the pancreas in a four-year old child. Texas J Med 28:464-467, 1932.
48. Smith WR: Primary carcinoma of the pancreas in children. Report of a case in a boy fourteen and one-half years of age, with generalized metastases. Am J Dis Child 50:-1482-1494, 1935.
49. Warthen RO, Sanford MD, Rice EC: Primary malignant tumor of the pancreas in a 15-month old boy. Am J Dis Child 83:663-666, 1952.
50. Grant GH, Percival PE: Carcinomas of the pancreas in a girl of 16. Presenting as carcinomatosis of lung. Br Med J 1:857, 1954.
51. Morlock CG, Dockerty MB: Carcinoma of the pancreas during the first two decades of life — Report of two cases. Postgrad Med 26:329-333, 1959.
52. Sanan DP, Singh A, Bawa YS: Pancreatic carcinoma in a girl of seventeen years. J Indian Med Assoc 50:579-582, 1968.
53. Tavassoli FA, Lynch RG: Occult adenocarcinoma of the pancreas in a 17-year old patient with immunosuppressed leukemia. Gastroenterology 66:1054-1057, 1974.
54. Warren KW: Nonfunctioning islet cell carcinoma in an 11-year old child treated by pancreatoduodenectomy. Lahey Clin Bull 9:155-159, 1955.
55. Becker WF: Pancreatoduodenectomy for carcinoma of the pancreas in an infant: report of a case. Ann Surg 145:864-872, 1957.
56. Wastell C: Malignant nonfunctioning islet cell tumor of the pancreas in a 14-year old girl. Proc Roy Soc Med 58:532-434, 1965.
57. Kissane JM: Carcinoma of the exocrine pancreas. Pathologic aspects. J Surg Oncol 7:-167-174, 1975.
58. Frabe WJ, Still WJS, Kay S: Carcinoma of the pancreas, infantile type. A light and electron microscopic type. Cancer 27:667-673, 1971.
59. Burns WA, Matthews MJ, Hamosh M, Van der Weide G, Blum R, Johnson FB: Lipase-secreting acinar cell carcinoma of the pancreas with polyarthropathy. A light and electron microscopic, histochemical and biochemical study. Cancer 33:1002-1009, 1974.
60. Stein ML, Rossi VC, De Almeida AMC: Carcinoma de pancreas em lactente. Apresentacas d um caso. Pediatria prat 33:75-82, 1962.
61. Hamoudi AB, Misugi K, Grosfeld JL, Reiner CB: Papillary epithelial neoplasm of pancreas in a child. Report of a case with electron microscopy. Cancer 26:1126-1134, 1970.

7. Pre-operative Evaluation of Pancreatic Tumors

KENNETH W. FALTERMAN and ISIDORE COHN, Jr.

1. INTRODUCTION

Pancreatic tumors are unusual in the pediatric age group. In reviewing disorders of the pancreas seen at the Children's Hospital Medical Center, Boston, over a forty-year period, Welch[1] reported only twenty-five patients with pancreatic tumors. Malignant pancreatic disease is even more unusual and, with few exceptions, is carcinoma. Moynan[2], in 1964, collected and reported 15 cases of pancreatic carcinoma in children. Welch[1] added 13 additional cases to bring the reported experience to 28.

2. SIGNS AND SYMPTOMS

Infants and children with pancreatic carcinoma present most often with signs and symptoms of abdominal pain and a palpable abdominal mass, not unlike the more common abdominal masses in this age group. Other clinical findings include: icterus, steatorrhea, anorexia, vomiting, anemia, weight loss, fever, melena and hematemesis. The 'usual' upper abdominal mass in infants and children should be evaluated in the time honored fashion designed to recognize the more common renal lesions, neural crest tumors, hepatic tumors, and lymphomas. Clinical suspicion or preliminary studies may suggest the presence of pancreatic malignancy. Various studies may help pinpoint the presence of the unusual pancreatic carcinoma in infants and children. These studies will be discussed in a sequence which might be used in investigating the patient rather than in any order of accuracy, desirability or historical development.

G. B. Humphrey et al. (eds.), Pancreatic Tumors in Children.
© 1982 Martinus Nijhoff Publishers, The Hague/Boston/London. ISBN-13:978-94-009-7617-7

3. IMMUNOLOGY

A much sought after goal is a highly selective and accurate serologic study to identify patients with early pancreatic carcinoma. In recent years progress has been made in identifying new tumor-associated antigens in patients with pancreatic carcinoma.

DiMagno et al. [3] measured the rate of excretion of carcinoembryonic antigen (CEA) into the duodenum under basal and stimulated conditions. They found CEA output rates were not helpful in diagnosing pancreatic carcinoma. Zamcheck [4] concluded that CEA studies can have a high level of accuracy in diagnosing pancreatic carcinoma. Sharma et al. [5] studied CEA activity in pure pancreatic juice obtained by peroral endoscopic cannulation of the pancreatic duct. Pancreatic juice CEA activity in patients with pancreatic carcinoma was significantly higher than in controls or in patients with pancreatitis. In this study no patient with a pancreatic juice CEA below 30 ng/ml and plasma CEA less than 2.5 ng/ml had pancreatic carcinoma. Kawanishi et al. [6] utilized an endoscopic technique to obtain pure pancreatic juice to study pancreatic function and CEA levels at the time of endoscopic retrograde cholangiopancreatography (ERCP). They believe the overall diagnostic reliability for pancreatic carcinoma can be increased with these combined procedures.

Gelder et al. [7] described purification, partial characterization and evaluation of a pancreatic oncofetal antigen. This antigen is found in fetal pancreas and pancreatic cancer tissue but not in normal adult pancreas, and is different from CEA and other known tumor-associated antigens. Pancreatic oncofetal antigen (POA) is found in the sera of most individuals, however, the highest absolute level and the highest frequency of elevated levels were found in sera of patients with carcinoma of the pancreas. Elevated levels of POA were seen also in the serum of patients with other malignancies as well as other benign conditions. Wood and Moossa [8] reported their prospective evaluation of tumor markers in 136 patients suspected of having major intra-abdominal pathology. At laparotomy 38 were found to have pancreatic cancer. Sera from this group of patients were assayed for CEA, POA, and alpha fetoprotein (αFP). True positive results for detecting pancreatic cancer were CEA, 48%; αFP, 33%; POA, 60%. True negative results for excluding a diagnosis of pancreatic cancer were CEA, 75; αFP, 71%; POA, 94%. A negative test for POA excluded the presence of pancreatic cancer with a theoretical error rate of 6%. Other investigators have reported the presence of additional tumor-associated antigens in human pancreatic cancer [9, 10].

In 1978 several investigators [11, 12, 13] reported their experience with use of the microleukocyte adherence inhibition (micro-LAI) assay. In this technique the patient's buffy-coat leukocytes are tested against crude membrane extracts of pancreas as a specific immunodiagnostic test for the presence of pancreatic cancer. The micro-LAI assay was able to detect specifically pancreatic cancer, and discriminate between pancreatic carcinoma, acute pancreatitis, other forms of cancer, and the normal state. These results suggest the micro-LAI may be a simple, noninvasive means of selecting patients with possible malignant pancreatic tumors who require further investigation. Tataryn et al. [14] used a tube LAI assay to study patients with various gastrointestinal cancers. In pancreatic cancer, 100% of patients with cancer less than 5 cm and without metastasis were LAI positive, whereas 29% were positive when the cancer was greater than 5 cm and had metastasized. Similar results were seen with other gastrointestinal cancers where lower stages of involvement had greater percentages of positive results. Obviously much more must be learned about the use of LAI assays, but it does appear this study may prove extremely valuable in detecting early lesions.

Investigation continues in an attempt to identify newer radioimmunoassay techniques which may be used to identify early pancreatic malignancy. Fedail et al. [15] reported high concentrations of lactoferrin in pancreatic juice from patients with chronic pancreatitis but considerably lower levels in samples from control subjects and patients with carcinoma of the pancreas. Soto et al. [16] noted abnormal secretory levels of immunoglobulins G, A, and M in patients with pancreatic cancer.

Though some believe tumor-associated antigens are still too fickle for population screening [17], recent progress with the micro-LAI assay and POA determination offer new hope for a sensitive and specific immunodiagnostic technique which may be used for screening of large populations in the future.

4. PANCREATIC FUNCTION TEST

Most pancreatic carcinomas are of ductal or acinar origin and therefore alterations in secretory function have been sought. Pancreatic function studies are based on direct or indirect measurement of certain components of pancreatic secretion. Some studies are quite gross and reflect only the malabsorption seen with advanced disease. Other studies are more selective and require endoscopic intubation of the pancreatic duct combined with stimulation by secretin or cholecystokinin (CCK).

Dreiling [18] has been a major proponent of the secretin test as a measure of pancreatic function and as a diagnostic aid in differentiating inflammatory disease, malignant disease, and normals. Based on volume of secretion, he reported a 95% positive rate for cancer of the head, 83% for cancer of the body and 81% for cancer of the tail. DiMagno *et al.* [19] and Malagelada [20] reported their experience with the CCK test which quantifies output of enzyme in response to 'maximal' doses of intravenous CCK. Pancreatic enzyme output was abnormal in 90% of patients with cancer of the head of the pancreas and 75% of patients with cancer of the pancreatic body and tail. Paminobenzoic acid (PABA) is split specifically by pancreatic chymotrypsin from the synthetic tripeptide N-benzoil-L-tyrosyl-PABA. Sacher, Kobsa and Shmerling [21] recently reported use of a PABA screening test for exocrine pancreatic function in infants and children. They measured urinary excretion of absorbed PABA which served as an index for exocrine pancreatic function. Recovery in patients with pancreatic insufficiency secondary to cystic fibrosis was very low with no overlap in the control group. This noninvasive method of studying pancreatic function may be useful in studying the child with suspected pancreatic carcinoma. However, one might suspect that in carcinoma only advanced disease and significant pancreatic dysfunction would result in the degree of malabsorption necessary for a positive screen. This simple noninvasive test may be promising and merits further investigation in younger infants and children.

5. CYTOLOGIC DIAGNOSIS

The early interest in cytology of duodenal aspirates for the diagnosis of pancreatic cancer diminished as other more productive techniques came to light. With the introduction of the fiberoptic endoscope and the ability to cannulate the ampulla of Vater, there has come a reawakening of interest in cell cytology as an adjunct to the direct visualization of the pancreatic ductal system. In reviewing the value of cytology in the diagnosis of gastrointestinal cancer, Vilardell [22] reported positive results in pancreatic cancer ranging from 42% to 79%. Kline, Joshi and Goldstein [23] reported abnormal cells in duodenal aspirates in 31 of 40 patients with pancreatic malignancies. There were no false positives in their 199 patients with benign lesions. Several investigators [24–27] have utilized cytologic studies on secretions obtained directly from the pancreatic duct at the time of ERCP. Positive results are increased to approximately 80% by direct aspiration of pancreatic juice. A newer technique of endoscopic rectrograde brush cytology has been reported recently by Osnes *et al.* [28]. They were able to obtain positive or suspicious cytology in 90% of their patients with primary pancreatic lesions. As is true with pancreatic secretory function tests, a higher probability of positive cytology exists with more proximal lesions.

6. IMAGING TECHNIQUES

Many imaging techniques are available to study the pancreas. Ultrasonography, computed transaxial tomography, abdominal angiography, endoscopic retrograde cholangiopancreatography, radionuclide scanning and abdominal thermography are techniques which have been studied for their role in the diagnosis of pancreatic carcinoma. Ultrasound has moved rapidly to the forefront of useful diagnostic techniques in the evaluation of children with abdominal tumors. Rapid technical progress in the available hardware has resulted in much improvement in image quality. Most institutions now have 'Real Time' ultrasound available and the near future probably will see some type of computed ultrasonographic technique. Braganza et al. [29] studied prospectively a group of patients suspected of having pancreatic disease. Ultrasound, computed tomography and isotope scanning were compared. In the control group, isotope scanning and computed tomography were shown to have a higher false positive rate than ultrasound. Ultrasound was thought to be superior for the diagnosis of pancreatic carcinoma. In a similar study Mackie et al. [30] reported 149 patients suspected of having pancreatic cancer who underwent ultrasound examination and later surgical exploration. A correct ultrasound diagnosis of pancreatic cancer was made in 81%, with 13 false positive reports. Ultrasound examination detected 94% of cancers confined to the head of the pancreas and 70% of cancers at other locations within the gland. They concluded that ultrasonic scanning can and should be used as an 'Early Screening' test for patients with symptoms suggestive of pancreatic cancer. With improvements in new hardware, better training of technicians and more expertise in ultrasound interpretation, ultrasound may become the most important imaging technique in diagnosis of pancreatic lesions.

Computed tomography is another noninvasive, painless imaging technique which has gained much acceptance and popularity in studying infants and children with abdominal masses. Newer generation scanners have reduced the radiation exposure for each cut and increased greatly the quality of the images. The persistent drawback to widespread utilization of CT scanning continues to be its extremely high cost.

In a recent general review of pancreatic imaging, comparing ultrasound and computed tomography Lee et al. [31] reported that neither CT nor ultrasound is clearly superior in all patients and in all pancreatic diseases. One recommendation is that ultrasound should be the method of choice in pregnant women and in children since it does not depend on ionizing radiation. Other investigators [32, 33] likewise have shown neither CT or ultrasound to be clearly superior to the other in pancreatic imaging. Braganza et al. [29] reported one drawback of CT was a high false positive rate.

6.1. Nuclear Scanning

When isotope scanning was first introduced it was thought of as a possible solution to the many-faceted problem of diagnosis of cancer of the pancreas. Subsequent experience has been disappointing in the hands of most investigators because of the inaccuracy of the technique, and because of the number of false positives. It is interesting that in the same year, one can find these two diametrically opposed views from different radiologists: '... The test was effective in screening and in detection; false-negative diagnoses were rare... A normal scan excluded pancreatic cancer with a probability greater than 95%.' [34] and '... A review of the clinical results exposes the method as unsatisfactory for general use... This dismal record casts grave doubts on the justification for including scintiscanning, as it is presently performed, in the category of standard procedures for the diagnosis of pancreatic disease' [35].

The obvious advantages of the method include the fact that it is a non-invasive technique which causes the patient little discomfort and, therefore, should be nearly ideal. The reality has been that the uptake by the pancreas of the isotope, ^{75}selenomethionine, is not sufficient to permit a high degree of accuracy in diagnosis, and there is overlap from adjacent viscera which tends to increase the diagnostic difficulties. Most believe the scintiscan may be helpful in isolated cases but probably is too nonspecific and insensitive to be of significant value when other more selective and accurate procedures are available. There still may be a role for radionuclide imaging in the diagnosis of pancreatic carcinoma with the recent introduction of multiplane emission tomography. Hall et al. [36] have shown an improved diagnostic accuracy and the ability to detect resectable tumors. Buonocore and Hubner [37] reported a preliminary study utilizing positron emission computed tomography after administration of C-labeled amino acids. Of 24 patients with known clinical outcome, there was one false positive and two false negative results. In normal subjects, they reliably identified the pancreas. With refinement of hardware, radionuclide scanning could become a more important noninvasive diagnostic tool in pancreatic carcinoma.

6.2. Endoscopic Techniques

Endoscopic retrograde cholangiopancreatography (ERCP) represents a combination of radiographic and endoscopic techniques. A variety of flexible fiberoptic scopes are now available in pediatric sizes and success has been achieved with ERCP in the pediatric age group. ERCP, a valuable technique to demonstrate pancreatic carcinoma, is most often combined with collection of pure pancreatic juice for cytologic diagnosis as well as pancreatic function studies [28, 38]. The performance of these adjunctive studies at the time the pancreatic duct is cannulated increases the diagnostic accuracy.

6.3. Angiography

Many times celiac and more selective angiography are indicated in children with an upper abdominal mass. This technique is invasive and requires considerable hardware, skill and expertise for optimal results. Sigstedt *et al.* [39] report an overall diagnostic accuracy of 93 % but also note with superselective studies an increase in complication rate to 9 %, compared with a 1 % rate for celiac injection. They found angiography to be a valuable method to diagnose carcinoma of the pancreas, estimate tumor size, and to predict resectability.

7. BIOPSY

Numerous biopsy techniques to study pancreatic lesions have been developed. These include wedge or needle biopsy at the time of operation. Newer biopsy techniques include percutaneous fine needle aspiration of pancreatic masses utilizing some guidance techniques, be it ultrasound, angiography, CT scanning or ERCP. More recently biopsy of pancreatic lesions under direct endoscopic control has been reported.

Biopsy of the pancreas at the time of operation is advocated by some and condemned by ohters. Those opposed to intra-operative biopsy of the pancreas by any technique cite a lack of diagnostic accuracy, the danger of fistula formation, a possible lethal outcome, and the value of the experienced clinician's acumen in making the diagnosis. Those who advocate the diagnostic biopsy claim that a radical surgical procedure should not be performed in the absence of histologic confirmation of the diagnosis, and report a lack of complications. There are relatively few papers that present comparative figures on the values and dangers of needle *versus* wedge biopsy under actual operative conditions. Isaacson *et al.* [40] reported a large experience with direct biopsy of the pancreas in 527 patients, and showed a high degree of accuracy and usefulness. Comparable expertise may not be found in all institutions, so not all workers can duplicate these results.

Other nonoperative biopsy techniques offer the opportunity to obtain a tissue diagnosis without laparotomy. This is performed with a fine needle (21–23 gauge) via the percutaneous route, and with some guidance mechanism [43, 44, 46]. Series involving several thousand aspirations have been reported and have not been associated with significant complications [41, 42, 43, 44]. Ferrucci *et al.* [45] reported one case of malignant seeding in the tract after fine needle aspiration biopsy.

Tsuchiya *et al.* [46] utilized a flexible fiberoptic endoscope to introduce a specially designed fine needle through the posterior wall of the stomach or duodenum to accomplish needle aspiration biopsy. A protuberance in the lumen of the GI tract helped in localizing the lesion. However, if no abnormalities were seen at the time of endoscopy, the needle could be introduced through the medial wall of the duodenum for a 'blind' fine needle aspiration.

Fine needle aspiration has earned a place in the diagnostic armamentarium in the search for pancreatic carcinoma. It is very sensitive, with 70 to 90% accuracy in reported series. False positive results are nearly nonexistent. Complications are unusual and as other nonoperative methods for palliation are developed these techniques may obviate the necessity for laparotomy in the patient with advanced disease. Because of the rare occurrence of pancreatic cancer in pediatric patients, radical pancreatic procedures should not be performed without prior histological diagnosis.

Several large prospective studies have attempted to evaluate the relative accuracy and sensitivity of a broad range of diagnostic tools [20, 47, 48, 49]. There is not unanimous agreement about the best test for the diagnosis of pancreatic cancer. Ultrasonography was reported by most to be quite sensitive and accurate. Since it is absolutely noninvasive, it is an ideal study to perform early in the evaluation of a patient with a suspected pancreatic carcinoma. It is even more ideal in the pediatric patient. Some authorities in pediatric diagnosis suggest that in the future ultrasonography, with many of the improvements to come, will in fact replace several of our standard diagnostic modalities used in evaluating infants and children with abdominal masses. ERCP achieved a very high rate of correct definitive diagnosis, and, when combined with pancreatic function studies and cytologic examination of pure pancreatic juice, the overall accuracy can be as high as 80 to 85%. There may be some limitations to these studies in the pediatric age group. Where instruments are available and expertise exists, this technique may be very helpful if a suspected pancreatic lesion is under investigation.

8. SUMMARY

Pancreatic carcinoma is an extremely unusual tumor in infants and children. In most instances the diagnosis is made by exclusion when other more common pediatric solid tumors are suspected. Where pancreatic malignancy was encountered and treated appropriately in children, survival statistics appear to be somewhat better than those in purely adult populations. The combination of an increased index of suspicion and utilization of the diagnostic tools discussed here should lead to earlier detection of lower stage lesions which could result in better survival statistics.

REFERENCES

1. Welch KJ: The pancreas (Ch 84). In: Pediatric surgery. Ravitch MM, Welch KJ, Benson CD, Aberdeen E, Randolph JG (eds). Chicago: Yearbook Medical Publishers, Inc, 1979, pp 865–868.
2. Moynan RW, Neerhout RC, Johnson TS: Pancreatic carcinoma in childhood. Case report and review. J Pediatr 65:711–720, 1964.
3. DiMagno EP, Malagelada JR, Moertel CG, Go VLW: Prospective evaluation of the pancreatic secretion of immunoreactive carcinoembryonic antigen, enzyme, and bicarbonate in patients suspected of having pancreatic cancer. Gastroenterology 73:457–461, 1977.
4. Zamcheck N: Immunology, tumor markers, and pancreatic cancer. J Surg Oncol 7:155–165, 1975.
5. Sharma MP, Gregg JA, Loewenstein MS, McCabe RP, Zamcheck N: Carcinoembryonic antigen (CEA) activity in pancreatic juice of patients with pancreatic carcinoma and pancreatitis. Cancer 38:2457–2461, 1976.
6. Kawanishi H, Sell JE, Pollard HM: Combined endoscopic pancreatic fluid collection and retrograde pancreatography in the diagnosis of pancreatic cancer and chronic pancreatitis. Gastrointest Endosc 22:82–85, 1975.
7. Gelder FB, Reese CJ, Moossa AR, Hall T, Hunter R: Purification, partial characterization, and clinical evaluation of a pancreatic oncofetal antigen. Cancer Res 38:313–324, 1978.
8. Wood RAB, Moossa AR: The prospective evaluation of tumour-associated antigens for the early diagnosis of pancreatic cancer. Br J Surg 64:718–720, 1977.
9. Schultz DR, Yunis AA: Tumor associated antigen in human pancreatic cancer. J Natl Cancer Institute 62:777–785, 1979.
10. Mihas AA: Immunologic studies on a pancreatic oncofetal protein. J Natl Cancer Institute 60:1439–1444, 1978.
11. Russo AJ, Douglass HO Jr, Leveson SH, Howell JH, Holyoke ED, Harvey SR, Chu TM, Goldrosen MH: Evaluation of the microleukocyte adherence inhibition assay as an immunodiagnostic test for pancreatic cancer. Cancer Res 38:2023–2029, 1978.
12. Taguchi K: Immunologic detection of primary carcinoma of the pancreas. Can J Surg 21:313–315, 1978.
13. Tataryn DN, MacFarlane JK, Thomson DMP: Leucocyte adherence inhibition for detecting specific tumor immunity in early pancreatic cancer. Lancet 1:1020–1022, 1978.
14. Tataryn DN, MacFarlane JK, Murray D, Thomson DMP: Tube leukocyte adherence inhibition (LAI) assay in gastrointestinal (GIT). Cancer 43:898–912, 1979.
15. Fedail SS, Harvey RF, Salmon PR, Read AE: Radioimmunoassay of lactoferrin in pancreatic juice as a test for pancreatic diseases. Lancet 1:181–182, 1978.
16. Soto JM, Aufses AH Jr, Dreiling DA: The pancreas and immunoglobulins. III. Secretory levels of immunoglobulins G, A, M in patients with hypersecretory disease, postkidney transplantation and pancreatic carcinoma. A new diagnostic test. Am J Gastroenterol 68:34–37, 1977.
17. Editorial: Tumour associated antigens: Still too fickle for population screening. Br Med J 2:535–536, 1977.
18. Dreiling DA: The early diagnosis of pancreatic cancer. Scand J Gastroenterol Suppl 6:115–122, 1970.

140

19. DiMagno EP, Malagelada JR, Taylor WF, Go VLW: A prospective comparison of current diagnostic tests for pancreatic cancer. N Engl J Med 297:737–742, 1977.
20. Malagelada JR: Pancreatic cancer. An overview of epidemiology, clinical presentation, and diagnosis. Mayo Clin Proc 54:459–467, 1979.
21. Sacher M, Kobsa A, Shmerling DH: PABA screening test for exocrine pancreatic function in infants and children. Arch Dis Child 53:639–641, 1978.
22. Vilardell F: Cytological diagnosis of digestive cancer. Am J Gastroenterol 70:357–364, 1978.
23. Kline TS, Joshi LP, Goldstein F: Preoperative diagnosis of pancreatic malignancy by the cytologic examination of duodenal secretions. Am J Clin Pathol 70:851–854, 1978.
24. Goodale RL, Condie RM, Dressel TD, Taylor TN, Gajl Peczalska K: A study of secretory proteins, cytology and tumor site in pancreatic cancer. Ann Surg 189:340–344, 1979.
25. Endo Y, Morii T, Tamura H, Okuda S: Cytodiagnosis of pancreatic malignant tumors by aspiration, under direct vision, using a duodenal fiberscope. Gastroenterology 67:944–951, 1974.
26. Hatfield ARW, Smithies A, Wilkins R, Levi AJ: Assessment of endoscopic retrograde cholangiopancreatography (ERCP) and pure pancreatic juice cytology in patients with pancreatic disease. Gut 17:14–21, 1976.
27. Olsen JH: Duodenal exfoliative cytology. Diagnosis of cancer of duodenum, pancreas, and biliary tract by exfoliative cytology. Scand J Gastroenterol Suppl 9:105–109, 1971.
28. Osnes M, Serck-Hanssen A, Kristensen O, Swensen T, Aune S, Myren J: Endoscopic retrograde brush cytology in patients with primary and secondary malignancies of the pancreas. Gut 20:279–289, 1979.
29. Braganza JM, Fawcitt RA, Forbes WStC, Isherwood I, Russell JGB, Prescott M, Testa HJ, Torrance HB, Howat HT: A clinical evaluation of isotope scanning, ultrasonography and computed tomography in pancreatic disease. Clin Radiol 29:639-646, 1978.
30. Mackie CR, Bowie J, Cooper MT, Kunzmann A, Moossa AR: Prospective evaluation of gray scale ultrasonography in the diagnosis of pancreatic cancer. Am J Surg 136:575–581, 1978.
31. Lee JKT, Stanley RJ, Melson GL, Sagel SS: Pancreatic imaging by ultrasound and computed tomography. A general review. Radiol Clin North Am 17:105–117, 1979.
32. Sheedy PF II, Stephens DH, Hattery RR, MacCarty RL, Williamson B Jr: Computed tomography of the pancreas. Radiol Clin North Am 15:349–366, 1977.
33. Husband JE, Meire HB, Kreel L: Comparison of ultrasound and computer-assisted tomography in pancreatic diagnosis. Br J Radiol 50:855–862, 1977.
34. McCarthy DM, Brown P, Melmed RN, Agnew JE, Bouchier IAD: ^{75}Se-selenomethionine scanning in the diagnosis of tumors of the pancreas and adjacent viscera: The use of the test and its impact on survival. Gut 13:75–87, 1972.
35. Bachrach WH, Birsner JW, Izenstark JL, Smith VL: Pancreatic scanning: A review. Gastroenterology 63:890–910, 1972.
36. Hall TJ, Cooper M, Hughes RG, Levin B, Skinner DB, Moossa AR: Pancreatic cancer screening: Analysis of the problem and the role of radionuclide imaging. Am J Surg 134:544–548, 1977.
37. Buonocore E, Hubner KF: Positron emission computed tomography of the pancreas: A preliminary study. Radiology 133:195–201, 1979.
38. Freeny PC, Ball TJ: Evaluation of endoscopic retrograde cholangiopancreatography and angiography in the diagnosis of pancreatic carcinoma. Am J Roentgenol 130:683–691, 1978.
39. Sigstedt B, Lunderquist A, Tylen U: The yield of angiography. I The yield of pancreatic angiography. Ann Radiol (Paris) 21:381–383, 1978.

40. Isaacson R, Weiland LH, McIlrath DC: Biopsy of the pancreas. Arch Surg 109:227–230, 1974.
41. Ihre TH, Pyk E, Raaschou-Nielsen T, Seligson U: Percutaneous fine needle aspiration biopsy during endoscopic retrograde cholangio-pancreatography. Scand J Gastroenterol 13:657–662, 1978.
42. McLoughlin MJ, Ho CS, Langer B, McHattie J, Tao LC: Fine needle aspiration biopsy of malignant lesions in and around the pancreas. Cancer 41:2413–2419, 1978.
43. Dekker A, Lloyd JC: Fine needle aspiration biopsy in ampullary and pancreatic carcinoma. Arch Surg 114:592–596, 1979.
44. Ho CS, McLoughlin MJ, McHattie JD, Tao LC: Percutaneous fine needle aspiration biopsy of the pancreas following endoscopic retrograde cholangiopancreatography. Radiology 125:351–353, 1977.
45. Ferrucci JT Jr, Wittenberg J, Margolies MN, Carey RW: Malignant seeding of the tract after thin-needle aspiration biopsy. Radiology 130:345–346, 1979.
46. Tsuchiya R, Henmi T, Kondo N, Akashi M, Harada N: Endoscopic aspiration biopsy of the pancreas. Gastroenterology 73:1050–1052, 1977.
47. Mackie CR, Dhorajiwala J, Blackstone MO, Bowie J, Moossa AR: Value of new diagnostic aids in relation to the disease process in pancreatic cancer. Lancet 2:385–389, 1979.
48. Fitzgerald PJ, Fortner JG, Watson RC, Schwartz MK, Sherlock P, Benua RS, Cubilla AL, Schottenfeld D, Miller D, Winawer SJ, Lightdale CJ, Leidner SD, Nisselbaum JS, Menendez-Botet CJ, Poleski MH: The value of diagnostic aids in detecting pancreas cancer. Cancer 41:868–879, 1978.
49. Wood RAB, Moossa AR, Blackstone MO, Bowie J, Collins P, Lu CT: Comparative value of four methods of investigating the pancreas. Surgery 80:518–522, 1976.

8. Surgical Therapy in Pancreatic Malignancies in Children

E. IDE SMITH

1. SURGICAL THERAPY IN PANCREATIC MALIGNANCIES IN CHILDREN

Although pancreatic malignancy is uncommon in children, the appropriate management is important because of the more favorable outlook in the child than in the adult. Tsukimoto estimates that about 60 cases have now been reported in the pediatric population [1]. From these cases it would also appear that with more thorough pathologic examination and an increased awareness of pediatric pancreatic malignancies, that some abdominal malignancies previously classified as undifferentiated may arise in the pancreas [1, 2, 3]. Because only a few operations have been performed for pancreatic malignancies in childhood, it is necessary to draw upon the adult experience in this field for principles of surgical management.

2. BASIC SCIENCE BACKGROUND FOR SURGERY OF THE PANCREAS IN CHILDHOOD

The pancreas arises in the fourth embryonic week from a dorsal and ventral anlage. The dorsal anlage is the largest and is the source of most of the islet-cell tissue. It is drained by the Duct of Santorini which may persist as the accessory pancreatic duct. The ventral anlage rotates to the embryo's right and posteriorly where it eventually fuses with the dorsal anlage. The ventral anlage forms the head of the pancreas and contributes the major Duct of Wirsung. The Duct of Wirsung usually joins the common biliary duct as the entry to the duodenum.

Several anatomical relationships complicate surgical removal of the pancreas. The head of the pancreas and duodenum share a blood supply from the gastroduodenal vessels which usually precludes excision of the duodenum. The route of the common bile duct through the pancreatic head in

G. B. Humphrey et al. (eds.), Pancreatic Tumors in Children.
© 1982 Martinus Nijhoff Publishers, The Hague / Boston / London. ISBN-13:978-94-009-7617-7

proximity to the Duct of Wirsung necessitates a by-pass for biliary drainage with pancreatic excision. Careful attention to preservation of the superior mesenteric vessels is demanded by their close proximity to the pancreas [4]. The splenic artery and vein course along the superior aspect of the pancreas so that preservation of the spleen with distal resections is difficult, but not mandatory.

In the surgeon's favor in the child is the usually delicate and unscarred nature of the pancreas and the adjacent tissue planes. Since chronic pancreatic disease is rare in childhood, the surgeon is more often dealing with a more favorable organ. Blood vessels, although of smaller caliber, tend to be more pliable and are not diseased.

Experience with the replacement therapy of the exocrine and endocrine functions of the pancreas has developed significantly in the past 20 years which facilitates the management of the physiological complications of partial or total removal of the pancreas.

Cancer of the pancreas has been provisionally staged by the Committee for TMN Staging of Pancreatic Carcinoma at the time of surgical exploration as follows [5]:

Stage I: T1, T2, NO, MO—No (or unknown) direct extension, or limited direct extension of tumor to adjacent viscera, with no (or unknown) regional node extension and absence of distant metastases. Limited direct extension was defined as involvement of organs adjacent to the pancreas (duodenum, common bile duct, or stomach) that could be removed en bloc with the pancreas if a curative resection was attempted.

Stage II: T3, NO, MO—Further direct extension of tumor into adjacent viscera, with no (or unknown) lymph node involvement and no distant metastases, which precluded surgical resection.

Stage III: TI–3, N–1, MO—Regional node metastases without clinical evidence of distant metastases.

Stage IV: TI–3, NO–1, M1—Distant metastatic disease in liver or other sites present.

The most common sites of metastasis in the combined series of Tsukimoto [6] were to the liver and to the lymph nodes. Although the most common nodal area was in the portal area, secondary deposits were seen in the mesenteric, periaortic and hilar nodes. Involvement of the spleen, although reported, is rare. Malignancies of the pancreas must also be differentiated from metastatic tumors which include neuroblastoma, malignant lymphoma, Hodgkin's and rhabdomyosarcoma of the biliary tract.

The operability or resectability of the pancreatic tumor is largely determined by the absence of invasion of the portal vein posterior to the body and of the aorta and inferior vena cava posterior to the head.

Pancreatic malignancies may be functioning or nonfunctioning; the former being very uncommon in childhood malignancies. Functioning tumors include those arising from the beta- or islet-cell associated with Zollinger-Ellison Syndrome. Nonfunctioning tumors may arise from any of the elements of the pancreas.

3. SURGICAL PROCEDURES EMPLOYED IN THE DIAGNOSIS AND TREATMENT OF PANCREATIC MALIGNANCIES

The following are the surgical procedures which are utilized in the surgical diagnosis and therapy of pancreatic malignancy.

3.1. Biopsy

Biopsy of pancreas has been the subject of considerable debate in the adult because of its accuracy and morbidity. The experienced pancreatic surgeon can be highly accurate on the basis of gross examination only. Operative biopsy is reported to have as much as a 35% false negative return [7]. When a tumor is detected within the head of the pancreas there is general agreement that transduodenal biopsy with a needle has proven to be quite satisfactory both for accuracy and avoiding tumor spread. Biopsy of the body and tail from the peritoneal cavity has not been as satisfactory.

There are three current techniques of biopsy: 1) needle biopsy, usually with a Vim-Silverman needle with 5% morbidity and 1% mortality; 2) open biopsy with scapel, usually a superficial shave biopsy, with 9% morbidity and 3% mortality in one series [7]; and 3) thin needle or aspiration biopsy with a 0% morbidity and 0% mortality and 60% accuracy of diagnosis. The complications of all types of biopsy are pancreatic fistulae, pancreatitis and intra-abdominal abscesses [8].

3.2. Whipple Pancreatoduodenectomy

The Whipple procedure, which is primarily employed for tumors of the head and neck of the pancreas, requires partial resection of the pancreas together with the duodenum and the distal stomach. A direct anastomosis of the pancreatic duct to the jejunum provides pancreatic drainage; an end-to-side choledochojejunostomy for biliary drainage; and a gastrojejunostomy for gastrointestinal continuity [9]. Vagotomy is recommended because of the ulcerogenic potential of the operation [10]. The operation has been employed in adults primarily for tumors of the Ampulla of Vater, and in these the five-year survival is given as 30% [11]. The Whipple operation leaves the patient with a potentially functioning portion of pancreatic tissue. Warren has reported a 12.5% incidence of diabetes and 21.4% incidence of pancreatic insufficiency in 89 adults [12]. An 88% pancreatectomy produces immediate diabetes in 100% of cases; a 70–88% resection—diabetes in approximately six weeks and a resection of less than 70% results in no diabetes [13]. The procedure is performed only when there is no evidence of metastases or extension. The morbidity in adults is 20–50% and the mortality approximately 20% [14]. The most common complication is a leak at the site of the anastomosis of the remaining pancreas to the jejunum. Overall in adults there is less than a 5% survival; although the results with ampullary malignancies is better. The average survival time is about 15 months. The procedure is limited in lesions of the body and tail, and is not satisfactory in ductal carcinomas which are often multicentric.

3.3. Pancreatectomy-Total

Total pancreatectomy, often with splenectomy, is applicable for malignancies of the body and tail of the pancreas and for multicentric ductal carcinoma. There is a high morbidity (50%) reported in adult patients and the mortality is comparable to that seen with the Whipple procedure [15]. In some surgical centers, however, the mortality has been lowered to 7% [16]. The total removal of the pancreas removes the danger of pancreatic leak and fistula. Increased morbidity arises from the problems seen with diabetes mellitus and with pancreatic exocrine dysfunction. In the total pancreatectomy it is necessary to remove the duodenum as in the Whipple operation.

More extensive operations which include dissection of the porta hepatis, celiac axis and the superior mesenteric artery, as well as removal of the portal vein beneath the pancreas with repair, and extensive nodal dissection have been proposed by Fortner in an attempt to improve results in the adult [17].

3.4. By-pass Procedures

In the patient with biliary obstruction and an inoperable or unresectable tumor, by-pass procedures are used. There is general agreement that if a biliary by-pass is needed that a gastrointestinal by-pass should also be performed. Such procedures are obviously palliative only.

4. SURGICAL EXPERIENCE WITH PANCREATIC MALIGNANCY IN CHILDHOOD

Surgical experience in pediatric pancreatic malignancy has been summarized by Tsukimoto for the Japanese literature and by Welch for North American and European literature, as illustrated in Tables 1 and 2 [16]. All the survivors in Welch's group (six patients from a total of 22) had a total pancreatectomy. Five of these were for nonfunctioning islet-cell carcinomas and the sixth was for duct-cell carcinoma. Tsukimoto reports 12 survivors from 23 patients. All five patients who had resection for pancreatoblastoma are surviving, while only one of eight resected for adenocarcinoma surviving. Only one patient is listed as having a pancreatoduodenectomy, while all others are reported as having had a resection. Whether a localized resection of a tumor of the body or tail with preservation of the proximal pancreas is a feasible alternative does not seem clear. At the time of surgery it is imperative that adequate frozen section examination be obtained to clarify the extent of the neoplasm.

From the reports of Tsukimoto and Welch, the need for an aggressive approach to the pancreatic malignancy in childhood is clearly substantiated. Adequate preoperative evaluation, and exploration in a surgical unit in which extensive pediatric surgical procedures can be carried out affords such a child the optimum chance for survival.

REFERENCES

1. Tsukimoto I, Tsuchida M: Pancreatic carcinoma in children in Japan — Review of the Japanese literature. In: This volume, chapter 9, pp. 149–157.
2. Welch KJ: The pancreas. In: Pediatric surgery, Vol 2, Ravitch MM, Welch KJ, Benson CD, Aberdeen E, Randolph JG (eds). Chicago, London: Year Book Medical Publishers, Inc, 1979, pp 857–877.
3. Moynan RW, Neerhout RC, Johnson TS: Pancreatic carcinoma in childhood. J Pediatr 65:711–720, 1964.
4. Frable WJ, Still WJS, Kay S: Carcinoma of the pancreas, infantile type. Cancer 27:667–673, 1971.
5. Pollard HM, et al: Staging of cancer of the pancreas. Cancer (March 15 Supplement):-1631–1637, 1981.
6. Tsukimoto I, Watanabe K, Jang-Bor L, Nakajima T: Pancreatic carcinoma in children in Japan. Cancer 31:1203–1207, 1973.
7. Schultz NJ, Sanders RJ: Evaluation of pancreatic biopsy. Ann Surg 158:1053–1057, 1963.
8. Evander A, Ihse I, Lunderquist A, Tylen U, Akerman M: Percutaneous cytadiagnosis of carcinoma of the pancreas and bile duct. Ann Surg 188:90–92, 1978.
9. Whipple AO, Parsons WB, Mullins CR: Treatment of carcinoma of the Ampulla of Vater. Ann Surg 102:763–776, 1935.
10. Scott HW, Dean RH, Parker T, Avant G: The role of vagotomy in pancreaticoduodenectomy. AnnSurg 191:688–696, 1980.
11. Longmire WP Jr, Traverso LW: The Whipple procedure and other standard operative approaches to pancreatic cancer. Cancer (March 15 Supplement): 1706–1711, 1981.
12. Warren KW: Complications of pancreatic surgery. Surg Clin North Am 6:683–698, 1957.
13. Yasugi H, Mizumoto R, Sakurai H, Honjo I: Changes in carbohydrate metabolism and endocrine function of remnant pancreas after major resection. Am J Surg 132:577–580, 1976.
14. Brooks JR: Operative approach to pancreatic carcinoma. Semin Oncol 6:357–367, 1979.

15. Cooperman AM: Cancer of the pancreas: a dilemma in treatment. Surg Clin North Am 61:107–115, 1981.
16. Levin B, ReMine WH, Hermann RE, Schein PS, Cohn I: Panel: Cancer of the pancreas. Am J Surg 135:185–191, 1978.
17. Fortner JG: Surgical principles for pancreatic cancer: regional total and subtotal pancreatectomy. Cancer (March 15 Supplement):1712–1718, 1981.

9. Pancreatic Carcinoma in Children in Japan — Review of the Japanese Literature

ICHIRO TSUKIMOTO and MASAHIRO TSUCHIDA

Primary carcinoma of the pancreas is mostly observed in individuals over 40 years of age, and has rarely been seen in children. A review of the world literature reveals about 60 cases of primary carcinoma of the pancreas in children 15 years of age and under [1–5].

In Japan, Suma [6] reported the first case of pancreatic carcinoma in a 3-year old boy. Since then, 23 cases have been reported in the Japanese literature [2, 6–26]. The uniqueness of this tumor is based on localization, age, and histopathological findings.

This report is intended to present a summary of the clinical findings of the 23 reported cases of pancreatic cancer in children in Japan. Details of the histopathological findings will be described by Horie in another chapter in this volume.

1. INCIDENCE

Kurihara [27] tabulated the incidence of pancreatic cancer under the age of 14 years and estimated the incidence at 0.01 per ten thousand of the Japanese population between 1937 and 1947, and 0.25 per thousand between 1957 and 1966.

According to the 1957–1976 editions of 'Annual Record of the Pathological Autopsy Cases in Japan' [28], the incidence of pancreatic carcinoma in the entire Japanese population is 2.4% of all autopsies and 4.6% of all malignancies. The incidence of pancreatic cancer under the age of 15 years in the entire Japanese population is 0.017% of all autopsies and 0.15% of all malignancies. This incidence seems to be higher than that reported in the world literature [29] (Table 1).

G. B. Humphrey et al. (eds.), Pancreatic Tumors in Children.
© *1982 Martinus Nijhoff Publishers, The Hague/Boston/London.* ISBN-13:978-94-009-7617-7

Table 1. Incidence of the pancreatic carcinoma in Japan

	Under the age of 15	All ages
All autopsy cases	82,987	374,428
All malignant disease	9,057	167,511
Pancreatic carcinoma	14	7,647

According to the Annual of the Pathological Autopsy Cases in Japan (1957–1976) [28].

2. AGE AND SEX

The ages of the patients reviewed ranged from 2 years and 6 months to the upper limit of 15 years. The average age at diagnosis was 7 years and 3 months (median = 6 years). Twelve of the Japanese children with pancreatic carcinoma were males, and eleven were females.

3. CLINICAL FINDINGS

The presenting complaints and pertinent history of the 23 patients are displayed in Table 2. The duration of initial symptoms from onset to admission ranged from 1 month to 11 months in 15 patients.

Symptoms, in order of frequency, were as follows. Abdominal distention or mass was noted in 15 patients. Abdominal pain occurred in 12 instances. Gastrointestinal symptoms such as vomiting and constipation were present in 7 patients. Four patients complained of weight loss and anorexia. Fever was noted in 4 patients, and one patient had jaundice. Two children presenting with Cushing's syndrome had ACTH-producing islet-cell carcinomas. No hypoglycemia was documented (Table 3).

Pertinent findings on physical examination are shown in Table 3. Abdominal mass was found in 21 patients. Hepatomegaly and splenomegaly were present in 3 cases and 2 cases, respectively. All the other patients showed abdominal distention, ascites, jaundice, emaciation, abdominal venous dilatation and tendency to bleed, either singularly or in combination.

4. LABORATORY AND ROENTGENOGRAPHIC FINDINGS

Hematologic data were not always described in detail, but a significant anemia (hemoglobin less than 10 g/dl or RBC less than 3.5 million/mm³)

Table 2. Pancreatic carcinoma in children in Japanese literature

Authors	Age/sex	Clinical findings	Surgery	Site	Microscopic diagnosis	Progression
Suma (1930) [6]	2 yrs, 10 mo/M	Abdominal pain and mass, weight loss	Exploration	Diffuse	Adenocarcinoma	Died 1 mo post-operation
Maeta (1950) [7]	15 yrs/M	Abdominal pain and mass	Exploration	Body	Adenocarcinoma	Died
Endo (1953) [8]	12 yrs/F	Abdominal pain and mass, jaundice, weight loss, ascites, hepatomegaly, fever	None	Head	Unclassified	Died 3 mo after Dx.
Furuya (1962) [9]	10 yrs/M	Abdominal pain, cough, anorexia, weight loss	Exploration	Unknown	Embryonal sarcoma	Died
Ogawa (1969) [10]	8 yrs/F	Abdominal mass, Cushing's syndrome	None	Tail	Islet-cell carcinoma	Died
Yajima (1969) [11]	9 yrs/F	Abdominal pain and mass ascites, anemia, anorexia, vomiting	Exploration	Diffuse	Unclassified	Died 1 mo post-operation
Utsunomiya (1968) [12]	14 yrs/F	Abdominal mass, vomiting, anorexia	Pancreatico-duodenectomy	Body	Adenocarcinoma	Died 6 mo post-operation
Furukawa (1970) [13]	2 yrs/M	Abdominal mass, hepato-splenomegaly, anemia, fever	Exploration	Body	Adenocarcinoma	Died
Hitai (1972) [14]	6 yrs/M	Abdominal pain and mass	Resection	Tail	Adenocarcinoma	Died 1.5 yrs post-operation
Tsukimoto (1973) [3]	4 yrs/F	Abdominal pain and mass, jaundice, bleeding tendencies, anemia, anorexia, vomiting	Exploration	Head	Adenocarcinoma	Died 1 mo post-operation
Endo (1973) [15]	2 yrs, 10 mo/M	Abdominal mass	Resection	Tail	Adenocarcinoma	Died 2 yrs 1 mo post-operation
	2 yrs, 6 mo/F	Abdominal mass	Resection	Tail	Adenocarcinoma	Alive 2 mo post-operation

Table 2. (Continued)

Authors	Age/sex	Clinical findings	Surgery	Site	Microscopic diagnosis	Progression
Toyota (1973) [16]	6 yrs/F	Abdominal pain and mass, splenomegaly, diarrhea	Resection	Tail	Unclassified	Alive 1 yr, 8 mo post-operation
Ikeda (1973) [17, 18]	3 yrs/F	Abdominal pain and mass, hepato-splenomegaly anorexia, weight loss	Resection	Tail	Islet-cell carcinoma	Alive 2 yrs post-operation
Ikeda (1974) [19]	7 yrs/M	Abdominal mass	Resection	Body, tail	Islet-cell carcinoma	Alive 10 mo post-operation
Nagao (1976) [20]	9 yrs/F	Abdominal mass	Resection, splenectomy	Tail	Islet-cell carcinoma	Relapse 2 yrs, 6 mo post-operation
Horie (1977) [21]	4 yrs, 11 mo/F	Abdominal pain and mass diarrhea, fever	Pancreatico-duodenectomy	Head	Pancreato-blastoma	Alive 16 yrs post-operation
	5 yrs, 11 mo/M	Abdominal mass	Resection	Head	Pancreato-blastoma	Alive 6.5 yrs post-operation
Nakayama (1977) [22]	3 yrs, 11 mo/F	Abdominal mass, jaundice, weight loss	Exploration	Diffuse	Pancreato-blastoma	Alive 6.5 mo post-operation
Ikehara (1978) [23]	9 yrs, 11 mo/F	Abdominal pain and mass, fever	Resection, splenectomy	Body	Cystadeno-carcinoma	Alive 2.5 yrs post-operation
Morita (1978) [24]	14 yrs/F	Abdominal mass	Resection	Unknown	Pancreato-blastoma	Alive 1 yr post-operation
Muchi (1978) [25]	7 yrs/M	Abdominal pain and mass, Cushing's s ynd	Resection	Tail	Islet-cell carcinoma	Alive 1 yr, 7 mo post-operation
Tsukamoto (1979) [26]	7 yrs/M	Abdominal pain and mass	Resection	Body, tail	Pancreato-blastoma	Died 1.5 yrs post-operation

Table 3. Clinical findings

Symptoms	
Enlarged abdomen or mass	15
Abdominal pain	12
Gastrointestinal symptoms	7
Weight loss	4
Fever	4
Anorexia	4
Polyphagia	2
Jaundice	1
Physical examination	
Abdominal mass	21
Hepatomegaly	3
Splenomegaly	2
Ascites	3
Jaundice	3
Emaciation	5
Abdominal venous distention	2
Anemia	5
Bleeding tendencies	1

was present in 4 of the 12 cases for which information was available. A leukocytosis over $10,000/mm^3$ was present in 5 of 11 cases. Accelerated erythrocyte sedimentation rate (more than 20 mm/hr) was noted in 5 of 10 cases. Elevated serum transaminase and serum amylase were noted in 3 of 8 cases, and lactic dehydrogenase was elevated in 2 of 7 cases.

Gastrointestinal series were performed in 11 patients, and an enlarged duodenal bulb with a widened duodenal loop was observed around the tumor mass. The angiogram of the abdominal aorta showed abnormal findings in 5 instances. Echograms were performed in 3 cases, and all showed solid tumor patterns.

5. TREATMENT

Of the 23 patients, 14 had resection of the tumors, including 2 pancreatoduodenectomies and 3 splenectomies. As shown in Table 4, the following tumors were resectable: 6 out of 7 tail tumors, 2 out of 4 head tumors, 5 out of 7 tumors involving the body and one case of unknown origin. Four additional cases had exploratory laparotomy only, in which all three diffuse tumors were included. In 2 of the 23 patients, no surgery was performed because of advanced stage of the tumors.

Various chemotherapeutic agents were administered, such as cyclophos-

Table 4. Site of tumor and resectability

		Head	Body	Tail	Diffuse	Unknown
No surgery	2	1	0	1	0	0
Exploratory	7	1	2	0	3 (1)[a]	1
Resection	12	1 (1)[a]	1 (1)	9[a] (7)[b]	0	1 (1)[a]
Pancreatoduodenectomy	2	1 (1)[a]	1	0	0	0
Total	23	4	4	10	3	2

[a] Pancreatoblastoma, one stellate corresponds to one case.
[b] Four of 7 survivors had islet-cell carcinoma.
( ) Survivors

phamide, vincristine, and mitomycin; few cases were treated with radiotherapy as well. Disappearance of obstructive jaundice, an increase of appetite, regression of the abdominal mass, and tumor necrosis at the time of autopsy were all interpreted as clinical evidence of tumor response to therapy.

6. PROGNOSIS

Of the 23 patients reviewed, 12 were reported post mortem. All the 11 patients surviving when reported had undergone complete surgical removal of the tumors. Of 13 cases reported since 1974, 7 were apparently doing well from 8 months to 16 years after surgery.

7. PATHOLOGY

An autopsy was performed in 5 patients. In the 18 other children, the surgical findings were available. The pathologic findings are presented in Table 2. The primary site of the tumor was head of the pancreas in 4 patients, body of the pancreas in 4, and tail in 8. The entire organ was diffusely involved in 5 (3 as diffuse and 2 body and tail). The site of origin in 2 patients was not known. Histologically, 9 cases were diagnosed as adenocarcinoma, 5 as pancreatoblastoma, 5 as islet-cell carcinoma, 1 as cystadenocarcinoma, 1 as sarcoma of the pancreas and 3 were unclassified carcinomas (Table 5).

Table 5. Histopathological diagnosis of the malignant pancreatic tumors in children in Japan

Pancreatic carcinoma	
Adenocarcinoma	8 (1)
Pancreatoblastoma	5 (4)
Cystadenocarcinoma	1 (1)
Unclassified	3 (1)
Islet-cell carcinoma	
Nonfunctioning	3 (3)
Functioning (ACTH)	2 (1)
Sarcoma of the pancreas	1 (0)

( ) Survivors.

8. DISCUSSION

Carcinoma of the pancreas is one of the very rare malignant tumors in childhood, and approximately 60 case have been reported in the English and Japanese literature. Of those, we were able to identify 23 Japanese cases. This may indicate that the pancreatic tumors in childhood are more common in Japan than in the other countries.

In contrast to the 2.3:1 male predominance in pancreatic cancer in adults, sex distribution is almost even in children with this tumor. Approximately 70% of the pancreatic carcinoma in adults develop in the head of the pancreas. But the primary site of the tumor among the Japanese children was more evenly distributed. The distribution in our case material was as follows: head of the pancreas in 4 patients, body in 4, body and tail in 3, tail in 7, while the entire organ was diffusely involved with tumor in 3 cases, and remaining 2 were unknown.

Morphologically, pancreatic carcinoma in children represents an unusual group of tumors which have not been previously identified. Except for the islet-cell carcinomas, the tumors sometimes showed admixtures of acinar and ductal elements which is a feature recently documented by Frable *et al.* [30] by means of histochemistry and electromicroscopy. They have applied the term 'infantile carcinoma of the pancreas', or 'pancreatoblastoma' [21] to this tumor.

As shown in Table 4, resectability and survival rate were high in the tail tumors of the pancreas: 9 out of 10 tail tumors were resected, and 6 of them were alive at the time they were reported. Interestingly, 5 of those 9 resected tail tumors were islet-cell carcinomas, and 4 of 5 were alive. These findings may indicate that endocrine tissue origin predominance in pancreatic tail carcinoma is the case in children as well as adults. Of the 4 head tumors reported, 2 were removed and the patients were alive. All 3 cases with diffuse involvement of the pancreas were unresectable. Of the 5 tumors with the unique histology defined as 'pancreatoblastoma', 2 originated in the head of the pancreas, 1 in the tail, 1 was diffuse, and the site of origin of 1 was unknown. Four patients were alive at the time of the report.

The cases diagnosed as pancreatoblastoma seemed to have a significantly better prognosis. But similar tumors may have been classified as adenocarcinoma or as unclassified by other reporters. Further clinico-pathological corrections should be investigated.

Because of the small number of the cases, the effectiveness of particular therapeutic regimens has not been demonstrated. However, there was evidence of therapeutic response to cyclophosphamide, vincristine and mitomycin C in several cases. All 11 patients alive when reported had undergone surgical resection and 7 had survived from 8 months to 16 years. Complete surgical removal should be the optimal therapeutic procedure for the pancreatic carcinoma in childhood.

9. ADDENDUM

After submitting this paper, Horie reviewed histologically 6 Japanese cases including our case (Tsukimoto, 1971) and diagnosed our case as pancreatoblastoma. Consequently, adenocarcinoma was decreased from 8 to 7 cases, and pancreatoblastoma was increased to 6 (2 of which were dead) in our review.

REFERENCES

1. Moynan RW, Neerhout RC, Johnson TS: Pancreatic carcinoma in childhood. J Pediatr 65:711–720, 1964.
2. Grosfeld JL, Clatworthy HW, Hamoudi AB: Pancreatic malignancy in children. Arch Surg 101:370–375, 1970.
3. Tsukimoto I, Watanabe K, Lin J, Nakajima T: Pancreatic carcinoma in children in Japan. Cancer 31:1203–1207, 1973.
4. Taxy JB: Adenocarcinoma of the pancreas in childhood. Report of a case and a review of the English language literature. Cancer 37:1508–1518, 1976.
5. Benjamin E, Wright DH: Adenocarcinoma of the pancreas of childhood: a report of two cases. Histopathology 4:87–104, 1980.
6. Suma K: Pancreatic carcinoma in childhood. Zika Zashi 357:179–192, 1930 (in Japanese).
7. Maeta T, Kikuta Y: Pancreatic carcinoma. Tohoku J Exp Med 45:26–28, 1950 (in Japanese).
8. Endo K, Sasamoto S: Primary carcinoma in young girl. Shinryo 6:571–574, 1953 (in Japanese).

9. Furuya A: Pancreatic cancer in 10-year old boy. Shonika Rinsho 15:320, 1962 (in Japanese).

10. Ogawa M, Iwase K, Furikawa H, Nagai R, Agei Y: A case of Cushing's syndrome caused by pancreatic tumor. Clin Endocrinol (Tokyo) 17:448–452, 1969 (in Japanese).

11. Yajima Y, Maeta K: Two cases of tumors of the digestive organs in children — transverse colon and pancreas. Shujutsu 23:1074–1078, 1969 (in Japanese).

12. Utsunomiya T, Kato S, Yamano N, Mikata A: Pancreatic carcinoma in children. Shonika Shinryo 31:112–118, 1968 (in Japanese).

13. Furukawa M, Mitsutake N, Tanaka N, Uchimura M, Masa Y, Tsuchiya R, Tsuji Y: A case of pancreatic cancer in infancy. J Jap Soc Pediatr Surg 6:65, 1970 (in Japanese).

14. Hitai H, Matsuoka S, Tanaka K, Takahashi T, Kikyo T, Okajima H: A case report on retroperitoneal carcinoma probably originated from the pancreas in a 6-year old boy. Shonigeka-Naika 4:811–817, 1972 (in Japanese).

15. Endo K, Kimura S, Shinomura T, Katsura S: Two cases of pancreatic cancer in infancy. J Jap Soc Pediatr Surg 9:543–544, 1973 (in Japanese).

16. Toyota N, Goto K, Kitayama T, Sugiura H, Aoki T: A case of pancreatic tumor in children. Acta Urol Jpn 64:985, 1973 (in Japanese).

17. Ikeda Y, Tsujimoto M, Okada T, Satani M, Okamoto E: A case of nonfunctioning islet-cell carcinoma of 3-year old girl. J Jap Soc Pediatr Surg 8:663–667, 1973 (in Japanese).

18. Kakudo K, Sakurai M, Miyaji T, Ikeda Y, Satani M, Manabe H: Pancreatic carcinoma in infancy — an electron microscopic study. Acta Pathol Jpn 26:719–726, 1976.

19. Ikeda Y, Itakura F, Kito M, Soda S, Hasegawa J, Tsujimoto M, Miyata M, Matsuyama M, Okada T, Takao T, Satani M, Manabe H: Two cases of nonfunctioning islet-cell carcinoma in children. J Jap Soc Pediatr Surg 10:297, 1974 (in Japanese).

20. Nagao K, Matsumoto T, Kondo K, Baba K: Prognosis of pancreatic cancer in children. J Jap Soc Pediatr Surg 12:108, 1976 (in Japanese).

21. Horie A, Yono Y, Kotoo Y, Miwa A: Morphogenesis of pancreatoblastoma, infantile carcinoma of the pancreas. Report of two cases. Cancer 39:247–254, 1977.

22. Nakayama M, Shimada H, Ssaki Y, Misugi K: Electron microscopic study of pancreatic cancer in children. Acta Pathol Jpn 66:164, 1977 (in Japanese).

23. Ikehara H, Fujita M, Arase M, Sakaguchi U, Tashiro M, Yokoyama I: A pediatric case of cystadenocarcinoma of the pancreas. Shonigeka 10:851–854, 1978 (in Japanese).

24. Morita N, Yamazaki S: A case of pancreatic cancer in children. J Jap Soc Pediatr Surg 14:1062, 1978 (in Japanese).

25. Muchi H, Oohira M, Ise T, Abe K, Adachi I, Kamegai T, Kawai F, Mori M, Kobayashi Y, Arima H, Nakamura T: A case of ectopic ACTH-producing islet-cell carcinoma in children. Gan no Rinsho 24:1343–1344, 1978 (in Japanese).

26. Tsukamoto M: Personal communication.

27. Kurihara M, Narai Y, Kiraide H, Suganuma T: Trend of age-specific death rates for cancer of pancreas in Japan. Tohoku Igaku Zashi 1:660–662, 1960 (in Japanese).

28. Japanese Pathological Society: Annual of the Pathological Autopsy Cases in Japan (No. 1-20). Tokyo, Japan: Japanese Pathological Society, 1957-1976 (in Japanese).

29. Wynder BL, Mabuchi K, Maruchi N, Betner JG: Epidemiology of cancer of the pancreas. J Natl Cancer Inst 50:645–667, 1973.

30. Frable WJ, Still WJS, Kay S: Carcinoma of the pancreas, infantile type. A light and electron microscopic study. Cancer 27:667–673, 1971.

10. Pancreatoblastoma. Histopathologic Criteria Based upon a Review of Six Cases

AKIO HORIE

So-called infantile carcinoma of the pancreas was highlighted as an entity in 1959 by Frantz in the first series of the Armed Forces Institute Pathology fascicle [1]. This particular case had originally been reported by Becker [2] two years previously. Since that date and until the present, the histogenesis of this particular tumor, if indeed it is a single entity, has been controversial. The two principal theories have been a tumor of exocrine derivation *versus* a nonfunctioning islet-cell neoplasm. In 1971, Frable and co-workers [3] described a tumor in the pancreas of a 4-year old female with histologic patterns including nests, cord-like structures, solid foci with a squamous appearance and a delicate stroma with thin-walled vascular channels. The ultrastructural features were quite suggestive of a ductal origin with acinar cell differentiation. Microvillous projections and membrane-bound granules were some of the more notable findings. These authors designated the tumor 'carcinoma of the pancreas, infantile type.' In 1974, two pancreatic tumors in children were presented at the 20th Annual Meeting of the Japanese Pathological Society [4] with similar features as those reported by Frable *et al.* The term 'pancreatoblastoma' was proposed to indicate the primitive or blastomatous nature of the tumor in line with the better known solid embryonic neoplasms of childhood, i.e., nephroblastoma, neuroblastoma and hepatoblastoma. Other authors have similarly equated the pancreatoblastoma and infantile type of pancreatic carcinoma [5, 6].

1. HISTOGENESIS AND PATHOLOGIC FEATURES

The author was aware of six pancreatic tumors occurring in Japanese children with have been reported in the English language and Japanese literature or as personal communications during a six-year period [7-12]. These cases have been summarized in Table 1. The children ranged in age

G. B. Humphrey et al. (eds.), Pancreatic Tumors in Children.
© *1982 Martinus Nijhoff Publishers, The Hague/Boston/London.* ISBN-13:978-94-009-7617-7

Table 1. Clinicopathologic features of pancreatoblastoma

Case	Authors	Age	Sex	Site	Size	Progression
1	Tsukimoto *et al.* [9]	4	F	Head	6 × 5 × 5	Died 30 days after laparotomy
2	Kakudo *et al.* [7]	3	F	Tail	15 × 5 × 5	Died 2 years after resection
3	Horie *et al.* [8] (1st case)	4	M	Head	11 × 9 × 8.5	Living well 20 years after resection
4	Horie *et al.* [8] (2nd case)	5	M	Head	7 × 6 × 4	Living well 7 years after resection
5	Sasaki *et al.* [10]	4	M	Whole	Unmeasured	Died 3⁴/₁₂ years after resection
6	Tsukamoto [12]	7	M	Whole	Unmeasured	Died 1½ years after resection

Addendum: Case #5: Autopsy report [11].

from three to seven years and there were four males and two females. Most tumors were quite large where measurements were available. Four of six patients were dead within four years of diagnosis although one of these was a post-operative death.

Histopathologically, the recognition of pancreatoblastoma has been predicated upon the presence of organoid structures, i.e., acinar differentiation and discrete squamoid nests. If the hypothesis is correct about distinctive tumors arising from the ventral primordia of the pancreas as opposed to the dorsal primordia, the aforementioned appearance may only apply to ventrally-derived neoplasms [13]. The composite criteria for the morphologic diagnosis of pancreatoblastoma are therefore the following based upon our and others' criteria. Acinar differentiation occurs in the form of alveolar structures with a lobulated configuration. The squamoid nests or cords consist of oval or spindle cells with a whorl-like arrangement. Keratinization is usually not present. The more primitive foci have a rosette-like, tubular or solid appearance. Small cells with scanty, pale or amphophilic cytoplasm are noted in these areas. Mitotic activity is not pronounced nor do the cells have anaplastic features. There is a PAS-positive and diastase-resistant material in the lumen of glands. Ultrastructurally, zymogen granules are identified in the slightly larger cells but not in the smaller, less mature cells (Figure 1). By light and electron microscopy, a primitive stroma of mesenchymal cells is prominent in some tumors. Other tumors may have a strikingly mesenchymal appearance at the expense of formed epithelial structures. The question is posed whether the former tumor should be considered a poorly-differentiated pancreatoblastoma. Two of the six cases (Cases #5

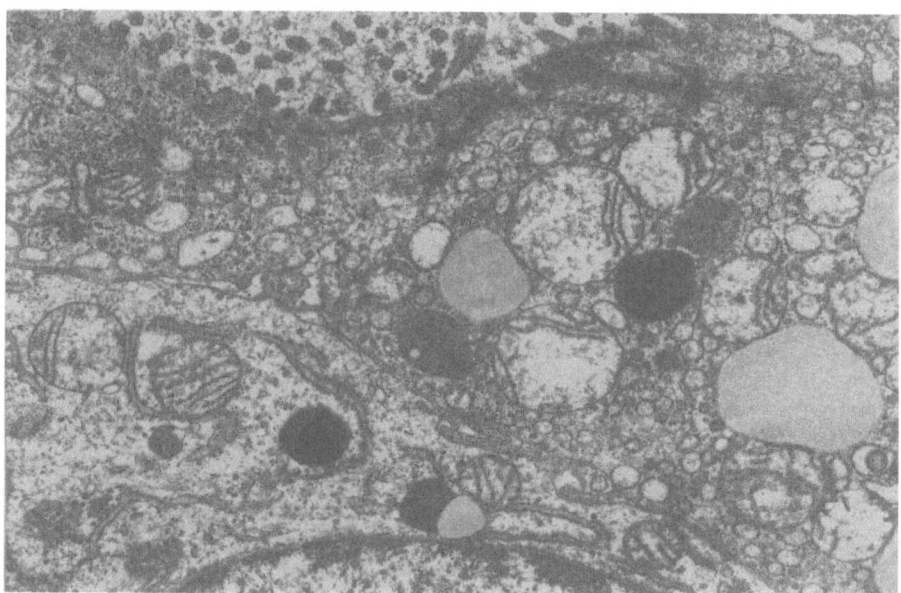

Figure 1. Electron micrograph of a pancreatoblastoma showing zymogen-like granules, glandular lumen with microvilli and junctional complexes (×13,600).

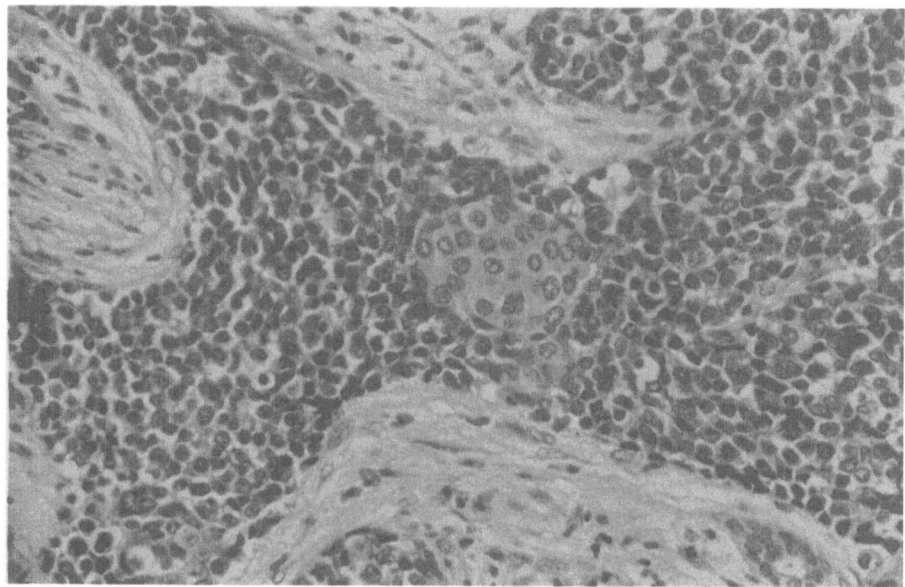

Figure 2. Poorly-differentiated pancreatoblastoma (Case #6) with squamoid areas, surrounded by the sheets of small cells, and poorly-formed glands (H & E, ×320).

162

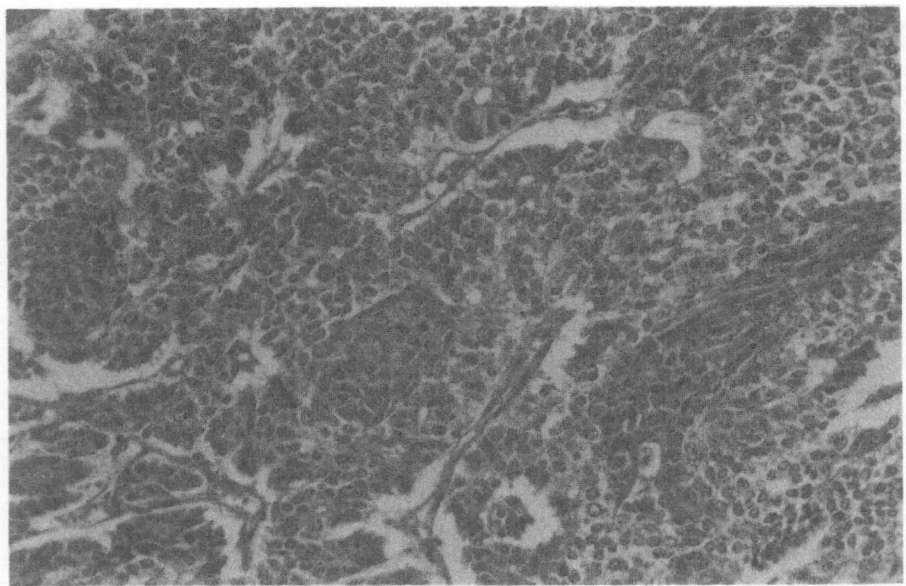

Figure 3. Well-differentiated pancreatoblastoma (Case # 4) with solid squamoid foci cords, and glandular structures (H & E, × 320).

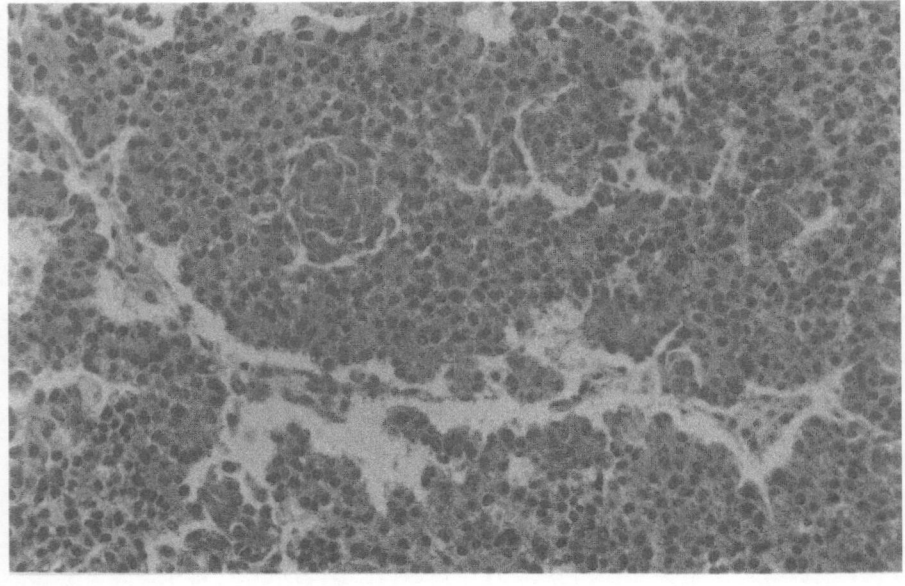

Figure 4. Well-differentiated pancreatoblastoma (Case # 1) with lobular arrangement, squamoid foci and small cells with acinar formation (H & E, × 320).

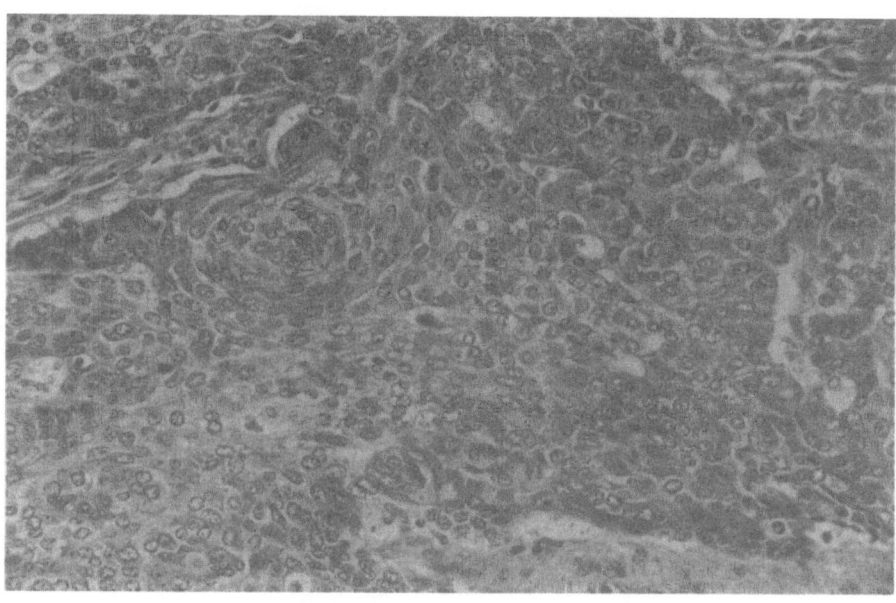

Figure 5. Well-differentiated pancreatoblastoma (Case #2) with medullary and tubular arrangement of cells (H & E, × 320).

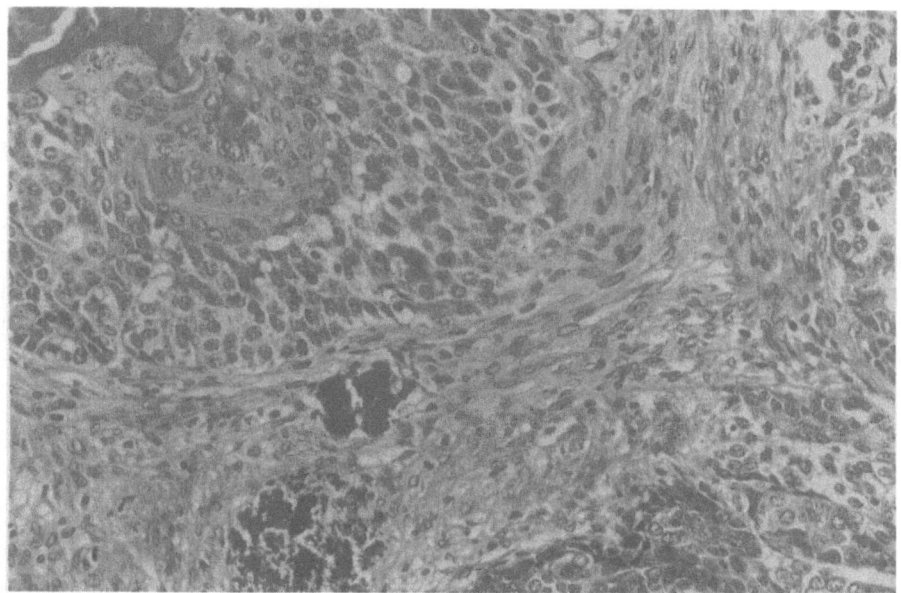

Figure 6. Squamous metaplasia of parenchyma and calcium deposition in the stroma (Case #2) (H & E, × 320).

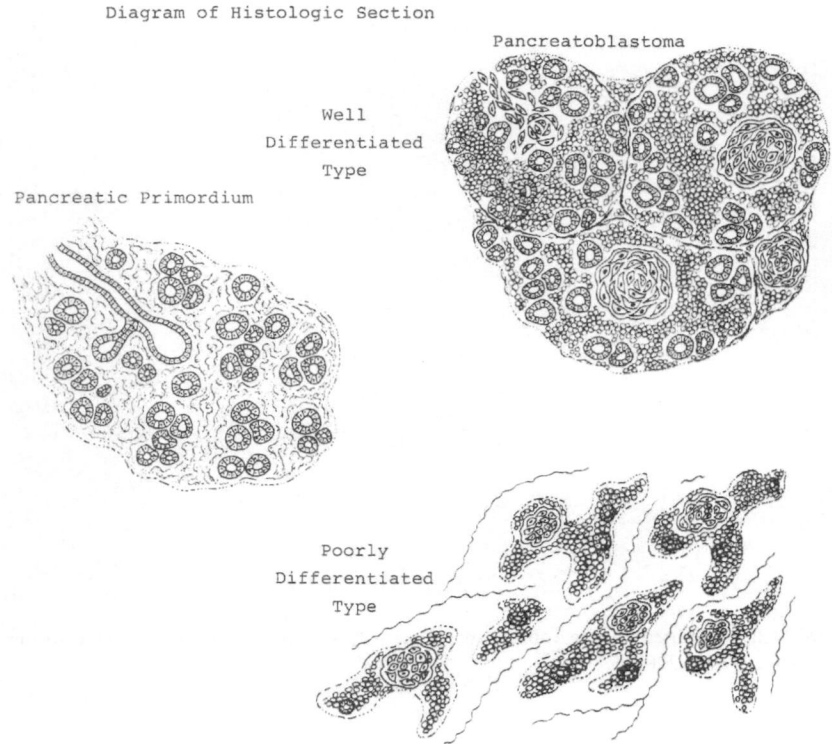

Diagram of Histologic Section

Pancreatoblastoma

Well
Differentiated
Type

Pancreatic Primordium

Poorly
Differentiated
Type

Figure 7. Diagnostic scheme of pancreatoblastoma.

and #6) were the least differentiated (Figure 2). At autopsy, one (Case #5) of these tumors had better-differentiated foci after irradiation and chemotherapy. This particular phenomenon has also been described in Wilms' tumors. The closest resemblance to the pancreatic primordia was attained in the remaining four tumors with the highest degree of differentiation in Cases #3 and #4 (Figure 3). Tubular, acinar and solid, squamoid foci were noted in Cases #1 and #2 as well (Figures 4–6). A comparison of these microscopic patterns with primordia of the pancreas is illustrated in Figure 7.

2. CLASSIFICATION

Taxy [14] proposed a subclassification of pancreatoblastoma into acinar and nonacinar types. His criteria are not strict since the organoid structures regardless of acinar or ductal differentiation are very similar to the pancreatic primordia. It is our contention since the pancreas is derived from sepa-

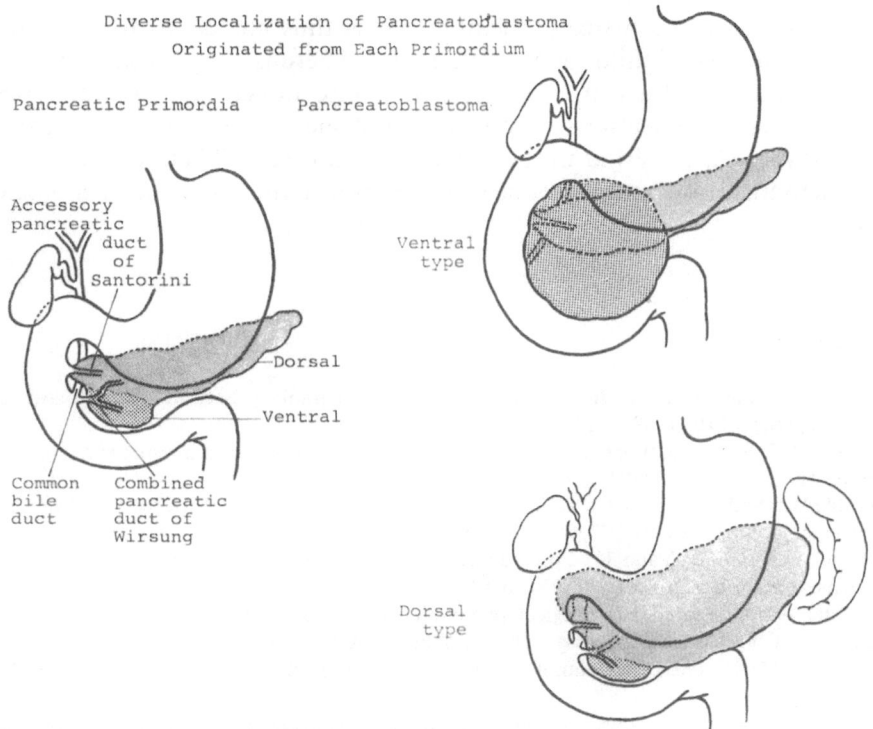

Figure 8. Localization of pancreatoblastoma based upon embryonic derivation.

rate anlage which fuse during development, that ventral and dorsal pancreatoblastomas exist. The features of a ventral pancreatoblastoma are an encapsulated tumor on the right side, dilation of the duodenal loop and a more favorable clinical course (Figure 8). Three cases (Cases #1, #3 and #4) in this study were classified as well-differentiated ventral pancreatoblastomas. In contrast, the dorsal type is a nonencapsulated tumor on the left side of the pancreas with an insidious clinical onset and extension into adjacent organs, liver metastases and an invariably fatal course (Figure 8). Two tumors (Case #5 and #6) were poorly-differentiated *dorsal* pancreatoblastomas and Case #2, a well-differentiated dorsal neoplasm.

3. CONCLUSION

Pancreatoblastoma is the preferred term for infantile carcinoma of the pancreas since 'infantile' is misleading from the standpoint of age when these children clinically present. This tumor recapitulates the organogenesis of the pancreas in its histologic features. It is thus analogous to the solid embryonic tumors of childhood in other sites. There is some suggestion that the pancreatoblastoma can be subclassified into dorsal and ventral types with prognostic implications. The histopathologic criteria for this differentiation have been reviewed in the context of six cases. Effective irradiation and chemotherapy may produce a transformation of the histologic features.

REFERENCES

1. Frantz VK: Tumor of the pancreas. In: Atlas of tumor pathology, Section 7, fasc 27 and 28. Washington: AFIP, 1959, p 132.
2. Becker WF: Pancreatoduodenectomy for carcinoma of the pancreas in an infant: report of a case. Ann Surg 145:864–872, 1957.
3. Frable WJ, Still WJS, Kay S: Carcinoma of the pancreas, infantile type. A light and electron microscopic study. Cancer 27:667–673, 1971.
4. Horie A, Kotoo Y, Yano K: Proceedings of the 20th Annual Autumnal Meeting of the Japanese Pathological Society, 1974, p 19.
5. Cubilla AL, Fitzgerald PJ: Surgical pathology of tumors of the exocrine pancreas. In: Tumors of the pancreas, Moossa AR (ed). Williams & Wilkins, 1980, pp 159–193.
6. Kissane JM: Pancreas. In: Pathology of infancy and childhood, 2nd ed, 1975, pp 320–344.
7. Kakudo K, Sakurai M, Miyaji T, Ikeda Y, Satani M, Manabe H: Pancreatic carcinoma in infancy — an electron microscopic study. Acta Pathol Jpn 26:719–726, 1976.
8. Horie A, Yano Y, Kotoo Y, Miwa A: Morphogenesis of pancreatoblastoma, infantile carcinoma of the pancreas. Report of two cases. Cancer 39:247–254, 1977.
9. Tsukimoto I, Watanabe K, Lin JB, Nakajima T: Pancreatic carcinoma in children in Japan. Cancer 31:1203–1207, 1973.
10. Sasaki Y, Nakayama M, Tsunoda A, Matsumoto S: A case of infantile carcinoma of the pancreas. Kanagawa Children's Medical Center Journal 6:216, 1977 (in Japanese).
11. Ooaki Y, Misugi K, Okudaira M: An autopsy case of infantile carcinoma of the pancreas. Kanagawa Children's Medical Center Journal 9:218–219, 1977 (in Japanese).
12. Tsukamoto M: Personal communication (a case to be published was operated in May, 1979).
13. Pattern BM: Human Embryology, 3rd ed. New York: McGraw-Hill, 1968, pp 387–391.
14. Taxy JB: Adenocarcinoma of the pancreas in childhood. Report of a case and a review of the English language literature. Cancer 37:1508–1518, 1976.

11. Solid and Papillary Epithelial Neoplasms of the Pancreas

JAMES E. OERTEL, GEOFFREY MENDELSOHN and JOHN COMPAGNO

An uncommon pancreatic neoplasm of epithelial origin, occurring most often in girls and young women, has been described in caucasians and orientals, and with disproportionate frequency, in blacks. A few men have been afflicted, but we have not encountered any cases in boys. Our earliest case on file is from 1927, a woman of 19 years.

Over the years the authors have collected data on 74 cases of solid and papillary epithelial neoplasms of the pancreas. Of these, 26 occurred in females between 10–20 years of age; 16 were caucasian, 5 were black, 1 was oriental, and in 4 the race was not stated.

The 11 patients aged 10 through 15 years (Group I) had signs and symptoms ranging from less than one day to one year in duration, with the majority two months or less. Four of the patients had sustained abdominal trauma; two of these four had symptoms less than one day, one had symptoms for four days, and one for one year. In the fifteen patients aged 16 through 20 years (Group II), four had symptoms of unknown duration, one had the neoplasm discovered incidentally during an operation for pelvic inflammatory disease, and ten were symptomatic for periods ranging from less than one day to three years (average about one year). One had sustained abdominal trauma less than one day prior to operation; one had sustained abdominal trauma seven years prior to surgery, but had symptoms only in the last two years.

Eight of the eleven patients in Group I had a mass and seven had pain or discomfort in the abdomen. A few had weight loss, malaise, or nausea and vomiting. Of the fifteen patients in Group II, twelve had a mass in the abdomen, eight suffered pain, and a few had weight loss, weakness, fatigue, or nausea and vomiting. One had no known symptoms (incidental finding), and in one case no history was available.

Radiographic studies, when performed, usually showed indentation or displacement of the stomach or duodenum and occasionally the kidney or the colon.

G. B. Humphrey et al. (eds.), Pancreatic Tumors in Children.
© *1982 Martinus Nijhoff Publishers, The Hague / Boston / London. ISBN-13:978-94-009-7617-7*

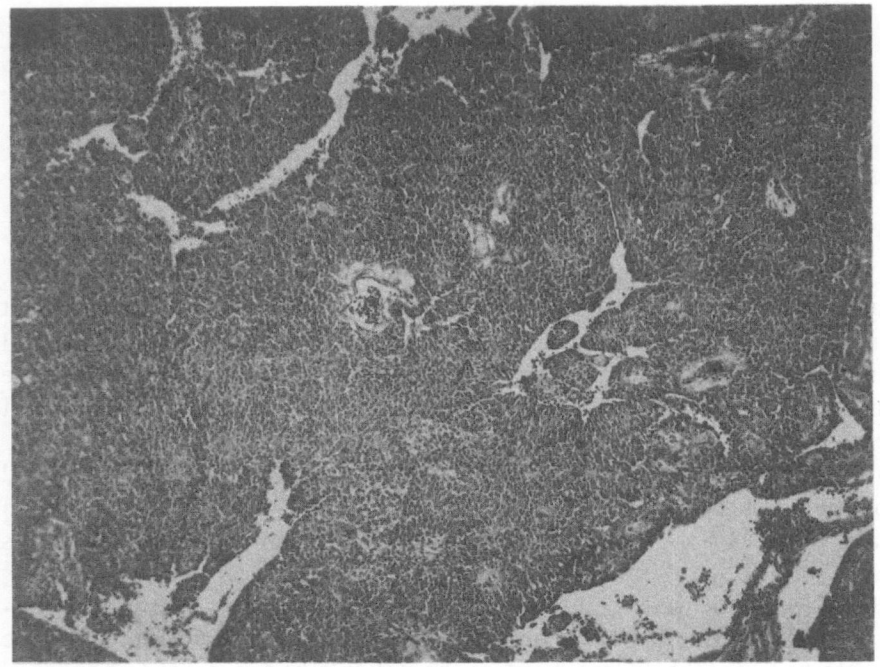

Figure 1. This typical neoplasm from a 19-year old woman had numerous solid foci (H & E, × 63).

In Group I six of the tumors were in the pancreatic head, two involved the body, and three were within or attached to the tail. In Group II three tumors involved the head, one the body, and eleven the tail. In one 13-year old girl with a history of abdominal trauma, the surgeon believed that there was laceration and hematoma of the pancreatic head; however, some tissue resected was later found to consist of clotted blood and neoplasm. She is alive 11 years later. In Group I the smallest tumor measured 3 × 4 cm, the largest 14 × 13.5 × 11 cm, and most were between 5 and 10 cm in diameter. In Group II the tumors were larger on average, the smallest approximately 6.5 × 5 × 4 cm (weight 74 g) and the largest about 13 cm in diameter (weight 1150 g). Most were encapsulated. The cut surfaces were pale and soft, often hemorrhagic, and often focally cystic or focally necrotic. The tumors were sometimes adherent to adjacent organs and soft tissue.

Operations were generally conservative with removal of gross tumor and adjacent pancreatic tissue. However, two pancreaticoduodenectomies were performed in Group I patients.

Microscopic examination demonstrated that the tumors characteristically

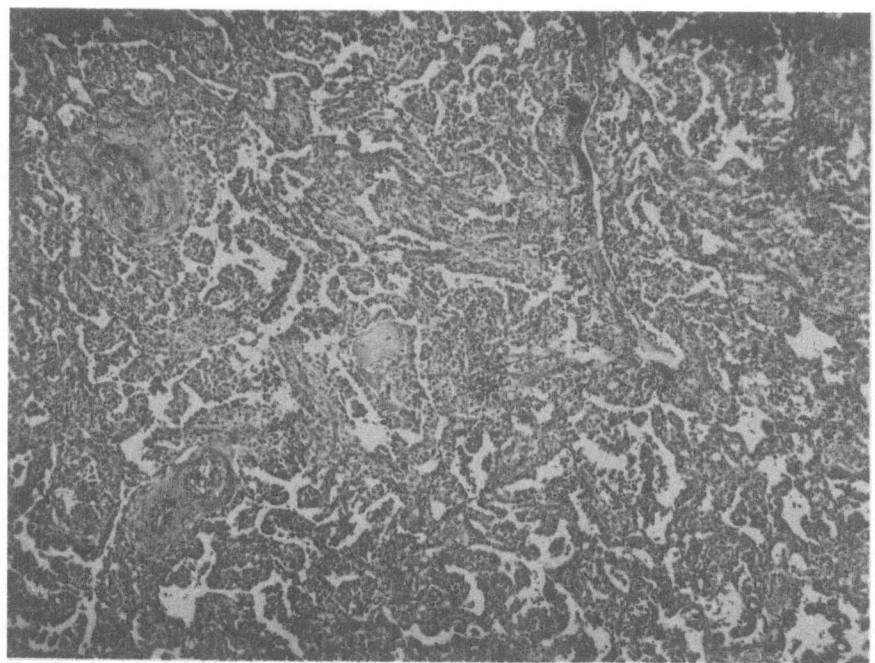

Figure 2. Numerous papillae were evident in part of the neoplasm (H & E, ×63).

had solid, papillary and cystic zones. Numerous small, thin-walled blood vessels traversed the neoplasm. Degeneration of those parts of the tissue farthest away from the vessels appeared to result in cystic change and development of the papillae. Hemorrhage and focal necrosis were common, and several tumors were almost entirely filled with blood. The neoplastic cells had lightly eosinophilic or almost clear cytoplasm and were ploygonal to somewhat elongated. Some cells were spindled. Nuclei tended to be small to medium-sized and ovoid, and chromatin was finely dispersed. Occasional cells contained eosinophilic, PAS-positive cytoplasmic globules. Foamy cells were occasionally present, as were crystals of lipid, usually in regions farthest from the vessels.

Some tumors infiltrated their capsules or the adjacent tissues, and rarely there was invasion of vessels, but such evidence of aggressive behavior was quite limited.

In nine of the eleven Group I patients follow-up from 2 to 22.5 years was available. All were alive, one with a peptic ulcer and one with diabetes mellitus. Of the fifteen Group II patients, one died suddenly three weeks after operation, two were lost to follow-up, and twelve were alive and well 3 to 15 years after operation.

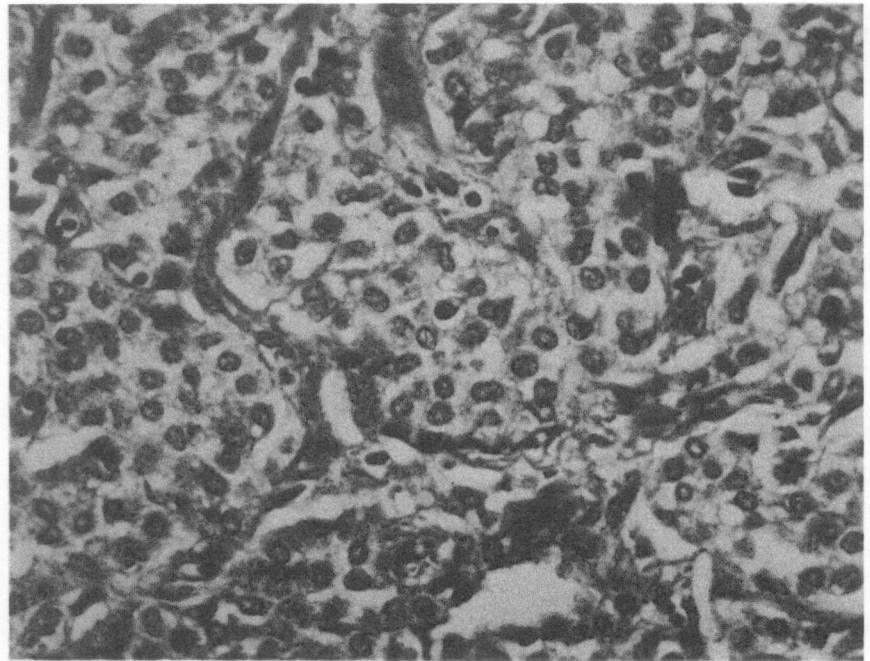

Figure 3. The cells have ovoid, slightly irregular nuclei and lightly-stained, occasionally vacuo-
lated cytoplasm (H & E, × 400).

Several patients over 20 years of age with this neoplasm have developed
peritoneal and hepatic metastases and at least one has died. This provides
additional evidence that the neoplasm is malignant, but not very aggressive,
and probably amenable to surgical cure in most instances. Long survivals
with apparent cures have been reported [1].

Several authors [2, 3, 4] have suggested that these neoplasms may be
related to the cells of the small ducts. However, the presence of immunoreactive somatostatin in a small proportion of the cells of one of the tumors
in an adolescent and a few of the older patients in our series suggests a
relation to islet cells. Nevertheless, the absence of somatostatin in most
examples, as well as of insulin and glucagon in all cases examined so far,
confirms that these are not islet-cell tumors in the usual sense. One histologically typical case, originally diagnosed as acinar cell carcinoma, which
we have studied by electron microscopy, contained scattered cells with
zymogen-type secretory granules. On the other hand, dense core neurosecre-
tory-type granules have been reported in another case [5]. It seems possible,
therefore, that these tumors consist of undifferentiated or uncommitted

epithelial cells, some of which can manifest exocrine or endocrine features.

Disclaimer — The opinions or assertions contained herein are the private views of the authors and are not to be construed as official or as reflecting the views of the Departments of the Army, Navy, or Defense.

REFERENCES

1. Frantz VK: Tumors of the pancreas. In: Atlas of Tumor Pathology, Section VII, Fascicles 27 and 28. Washington, DC: Armed Forces Institute of Pathology, 1959, pp 32–33.
2. Compagno J, Oertel JE, Kremzar M: Solid and papillary epithelial neoplasm of the pancreas, probably of small duct origin: a clinicopathologic study of 52 cases. Lab Invest 40:248–249, 1979.
3. Glenner GG, Mallory GK: The cystadenoma and related nonfunctional tumors of the pancreas. Pathogenesis, classification, and significance. Cancer 9:980–996, 1956.
4. Hamoudi AB, Misugi K, Grosfeld JL, Reiner CB: Papillary epithelial neoplasm of pancreas in a child. Report of a case with electron microscopy. Cancer 26:1126–1134, 1970.
5. Schlosnagle DC, Campbell WG Jr: The papillary and solid neoplasm of the pancreas: a report of two cases with electron microscopy, one containing neurosecretory granules. Cancer 47:2603–2610, 1981.

12. Ectopic Cushing's Syndrome in an Adolescent

JAMES H. SCHMIDT and THEODORE J. PYSHER

The islet cells of the pancreas normally produce a number of hormones and there is evidence to suggest that the precursors from which these cells arise have the potential to produce additional humorally active substances during neoplastic transformation [1]. Pancreatic tumors, especially islet-cell tumors, are uncommon during childhood and adolescence. In this paper we report an adolescent with Cushing's syndrome and hypergastrinemia which resulted from a pancreatic islet-cell tumor.

1. CASE REPORT

The patient was a 19-year old half American Indian half black woman who was referred for evaluation of Cushing's syndrome. She had been well until nine months prior to referral when she began to experience vague abdominal pain and generalized weakness. By six months prior to referral a change in her physical appearance was noted, characterized by weight gain, facial fullness, development of violaceous striae, hyperpigmented skin folds and hirsutism. Evaluation at another institution revealed increased urinary excretion of 17-hydroxysteroids and 17-ketosteroids and absence of X-ray evidence of any sellar abnormality. During that hospitalization, the patient developed melena and anemia and was noted to have esophagitis and a duodenal ulcer at endoscopy. She was then referred for further evaluation.

Examination revealed a Cushingoid woman whose somatic changes were striking when compared with relatively recent photographs. Vital signs were normal. Hirsutism, prominent axillary and abdominal striae and hyperpigmented skin folds were present. The remainder of the examination was generally normal. The stool was negative for occult blood.

Laboratory evaluation revealed a hemoglobin of 10.9 g per 100 ml, and a

G. B. Humphrey et al. (eds.), Pancreatic Tumors in Children.
© 1982 Martinus Nijhoff Publishers, The Hague / Boston / London. ISBN-13:978-94-009-7617-7

white blood cell count of 17,900 per cubic millimeter. Serum sodium was 143 meq, potassium was 4.4 meq, chloride was 101 meq, and carbon dioxide was 29 meq per liter. The urea nitrogen was 16 mg, creatinine was 1.0 mg, glucose was 116 mg, calcium was 9.2 mg, and phosphorous was 3.9 mg per 100 ml. Dexamethasone suppression tests on two occasions failed to show conclusive inhibition of urinary excretion of either 17-hydroxysteroids or 17-ketosteroids. Plasma cortisol levels also showed no uniform response to testing and ranged from 24 to 34 µg per 100 ml without diurnal variation. Urinary free cortisol excretion, although always in excess of the normal range (10 to 34 µg per 24 hours), did fall from 1193 to 122 µg per 24 hours during one dexamethasone suppression test. Plasma ACTH levels ranged from 136 to 64 pg per ml (normal 25 to 100).

Gastric analysis revealed a basal acid output of 36.1 meq per hour (normal 0 to 10), and a maximum stimulated output of 73.6 meq per hour (normal 10 to 40) while serum gastrin levels were consistently elevated, ranging from 1,015 to 1,564 pg per ml (normal 55 to 150).

Skull radiographs, sellar tomography, and computerized axial tomography (CT) of the head revealed no evidence of a pituitary lesion. A chest X-ray was normal. Computerized tomography of the abdomen revealed slight bilateral enlargement of the adrenal glands and diffuse thickening of the pancreas. No mass lesions were detected. A sulfur colloid nuclear scan of the liver and spleen was unremarkable and an iodocholesterol adrenal scan suggested bilateral hyperplasia. Selective visceral angiography revealed a vascular abnormality in the region of the head of the pancreas but was otherwise normal.

At laparatomy bilateral adrenal enlargement was confirmed. The liver was normal by gross examination as were most other abdominal viscera, but a 3 cm by 3 cm firm mass was identified in the head of the pancreas adjacent to the second portion of the duodenum. A frozen section was interpreted as malignant tumor and a pancreaticoduodenectomy and truncal vagotomy were performed. The patient's operative and immediate post-operative course were uneventful except for mild hyperglycemia. On the third post-operative day mild hypertension was evident and that evening the patient abruptly developed a severe headache and rapidly became lethargic then comatose. A cranial CT scan revealed gross intracerebral and intraventricular hemorrhage. The patient subsequently expired and the family denied permission for postmortem examination. A plasma ACTH level which had been obtained on the first day after surgery was less than 5 pg per ml.

Gross examination of the surgical specimen revealed a white fibrous mass in the head of the pancreas measuring 6.0 by 4.0 by 3.5 cm which was adherent to the overlying intestine. The intestine showed thickening and

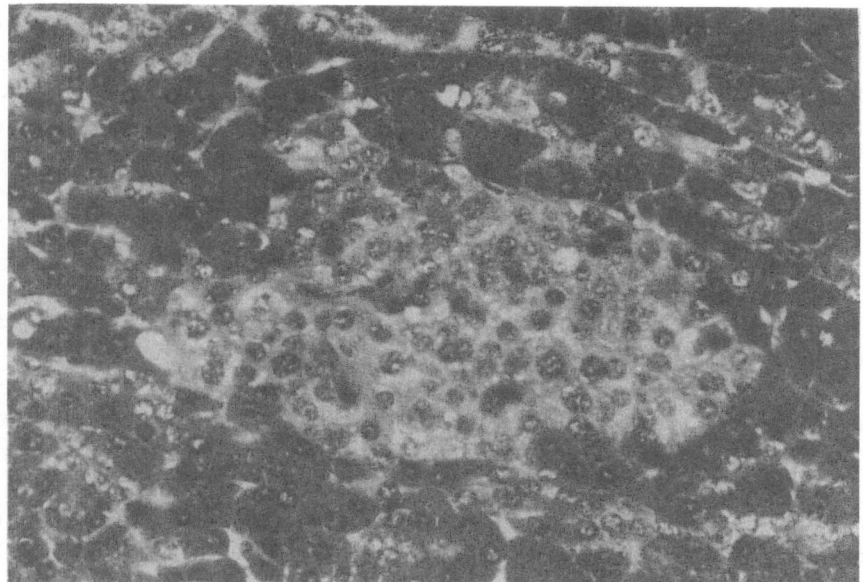

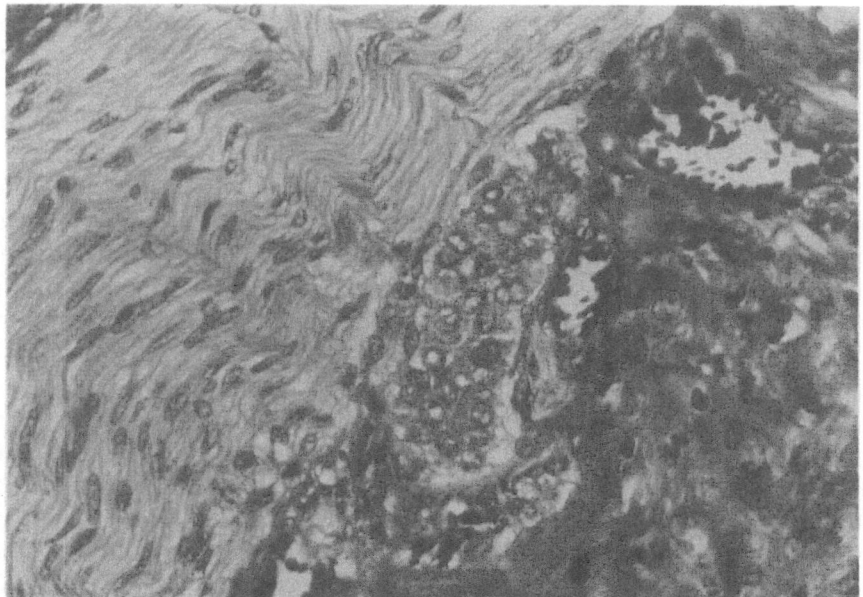

Figure 1. Comparable photomicrographs of tumor cells invading a perineural sheath (A) and a normal islet (B) demonstrate the histologic similarity of malignant cells to normal islet elements (H & E, ×65).

retraction of mucosal folds immediately above the mass and a section through the area showed protrusion of tissue through the muscular layers to the submucosa. The remaining pancreas was pink-tan in color and showed a normal lobulated architecture except for its proximal portion which revealed a firm gray-white parenchyma which merged imperceptibly with the tumor mass. Histologically, at the transition between pancreas and tumor, broad bands of fibrous tissue separated the parenchyma into nodules containing recognizable islets and acini admixed with a proliferation of islet cells and nodules of tumor characterized by nests and cords of small polyhedral cells with small amounts of eosinophilic cytoplasm and central, generally regular, nuclei with a finely stippled chromatin pattern (Figure 1). Focally, tumor cells were noted within blood vessels, lymphatics, and perineural sheaths. Ultrastructurally, the tumor cells contained numerous round to polyhedral electron-dense membrane-bound cytoplasmic granules ranging in size from 0.3 to 0.8 microns (Figure 2). A few dilated cisternae of rough endoplasmic reticulum were also present. The final pathologic impression was malignant islet-cell tumor.

2. DISCUSSION

This adolescent woman developed clinical features of Cushing's syndrome. Clinical and laboratory investigations confirmed the presence of elevated cortisol levels which did not respond to attempted manipulation of the hypothalamic–pituitary–adrenal axis. Normal radiographic examination of the sella in association with the elevated plasma ACTH levels pointed to 'ectopic' production of ACTH. The patient also manifested peptic ulcer disease with excessive gastric acid production and marked hypergastrinemia, suggesting the presence of a gastrinoma. The possibility that the entire clinical syndrome was produced by a functioning pancreatic tumor was supported by the pancreatic angiogram and eventually by the findings at surgery. The dramatic drop in the plasma ACTH level after removal of the tumor implies the presence of a causal relationship.

The histologic features of the tumor, particularly its tendency to aggregate in nests and cords, and the regular round nuclei with a finely stippled chromatin pattern are characteristic of islet-cell tumors. The presence of cells within blood vessels and lymphatics implies malignant behavior. The identity of the cell of origin can often be determined by the ultrastructural appearance of the secretory granules, but in many instances cells are poorly granulated or, as in the present case, contain only small granules [2]. Such granules are diagnostic of an endocrine tumor and consistent with a tumor secreting ACTH, but the large number of 'small granule' endocrine pan-

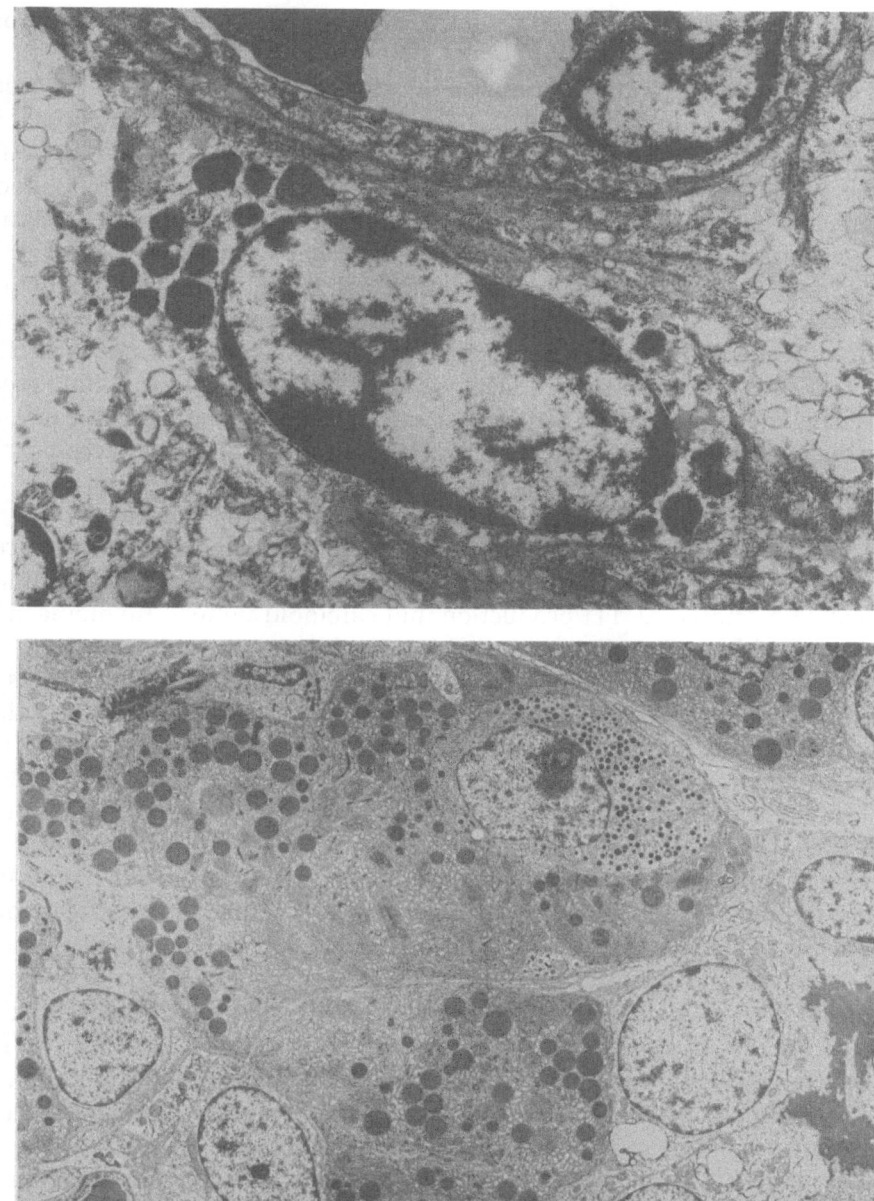

Figure 2. (A) A poorly-preserved tumor cell adjacent to a capillary contains several large electron-dense granules up to 800 nm in diameter (× 13,000); (B) A portion of pancreas near the tumor shows granular (300 to 500 nm) and agranular cells interspersed among exocrine cells (characterized by abundant rough endoplasmic reticulum and numerous primary and secondary lysosomes) (× 9,750).

creatic tumors necessitates some form of functional evaluation for more definitive diagnosis.

Pancreatic tumors are uncommon in childhood, and when they occur adenocarcinoma predominates. Fifteen cases of pancreatic carcinoma in individuals fifteen years of age or younger were described in 1964 and only three were felt to be islet-cell tumors [3]. Additional cases of childhood pancreatic cancer have been reported [4] but islet-cell tumors are primarily tumors of adulthood with the mean age at diagnosis being 44 years [5].

Cushing's syndrome may be due to hypothalamic-pituitary dysfunction with excessive ACTH secretion, may be due to autonomous function of neoplastic adrenal tissue, or may result from adrenal stimulation by ACTH or ACTH-like substances produced in 'ectopic' sites. During childhood, adrenal lesions, especially adrenal cortical cancer, are the leading cause of Cushing's syndrome [6], whereas in adults pituitary disorders account for about two thirds of the cases [7].

Among the numerous reported ectopic hormone syndromes, ectopic ACTH production is one of the more completely characterized. Oat-cell carcinoma of the lung is the most frequently encountered disorder associated with ectopic ACTH production, but carcinoid tumors, thymoma, and pancreatic islet-cell tumors comprise a significant portion as well [8, 9]. Interestingly, even when oat-cell carcinoma produces ACTH, rarely is it associated with clinical Cushing's syndrome, whereas patients with other ACTH-secreting neoplasms more frequently manifest the syndrome [9, 10]. The explanation for the discrepancy may lie in the possibility that immunologic detection of ACTH within the tumor or within the circulation does not directly imply bioactivity.

Hypokalemia and metabolic alkalosis are common chemical manifestations of the ectopic ACTH syndrome and are actually more frequently encountered than clinical Cushing's syndrome. Their absence in the present case was noteworthy and might have led some to question the actual presence of the syndrome [8]. Hyperpigmentation, which was evident in this patient, occurs in approximately 25 percent of patients with ectopic ACTH production [10]. Its occurrence is felt to be due in part to the elaboration of β-lipotropin along with ACTH from a common precursor molecule, since it does not occur in simple cases of hypercortisolism [7].

The patient also manifested the clinical effects of excessive gastric acid secretion and was noted to have very high circulating gastrin levels, however other features of the Zollinger-Ellison syndrome were not present. Gastrin-producing islet-cell tumors are well recognized, further, islet-cell tumors which secrete multiple hormones are well described. One of the earlier well-documented reports of multiple hormone secretion by an islet-cell tumor described a patient similar to the one reported herein. That patient's tumor produced ACTH, MSH, and gastrin and resulted in Cushing's syndrome, hyperpigmentation, and duodenal ulceration [11].

The optimum management for patients with islet-cell tumors has not been established. Surgery appears to provide the only chance for cure, but complete excision is unlikely since metastatic disease is present at the time of diagnosis in as many as 85 percent of patients [5]. Combination chemotherapy directed at complete tumor destruction has not been successful, but palliative therapy is available for clinical manifestations. Surgical or medical adrenalectomy has been utilized to control the problem of hypercortisolism; gastrectomy or cimetidine-induced inhibition of gastric acid secretion has been used for management of hypergastrinemia and peptic ulceration. It remains, however, that better therapy is clearly needed for all of the islet-cell tumors since the mean survival from time of diagnosis is only 2.8 years [5].

REFERENCES

1. Modlin IM: Endocrine Tumors of the Pancreas. Surg Gynecol Obstet 149:751–769, 1979.
2. Larsson L-I: Endocrine Pancreatic Tumors. Hum Pathol 9:401–416, 1978.
3. Moynan RW, Neerhout RC, Johnson TS: Pancreatic Carcinoma in Childhood. J Pediatr 65:711–720, 1964.
4. Tsukimoto I, Watanabe K, Lin J-B, Nakajima T: Pancreatic Carcinoma in Children in Japan. Cancer 31:1203–1207, 1973.
5. Cubilla AL, Hajdu SI: Islet Cell Carcinoma of the Pancreas. Arch Pathol 99:204–207, 1975.
6. Gilbert MG, Cleveland WW: Cushing's Syndrome in Infancy. Pediatrics 46:217–229, 1970.
7. Gold EM: The Cushing's Syndromes: Changing Views of Diagnosis and Treatment. Ann Intern Med 90:829–844, 1979.
8. Azzopardi JG, Williams ED: Pathology of 'Nonendocrine' Tumors Associated with Cushing's Syndrome. Cancer 22:274–286, 1968.
9. Imura H: Ectopic Hormone Syndromes. Clin Endocrinol Metab 9:235–260, 1980.
10. Imura H, Matsukura S, Yamamoto H, Hirata Y, Nakai Y, Endo J, Tanaka A, Nakamura M: Studies on Ectopic ACTH-Producing Tumors. II. Clinical and Biochemical Features of 30 Cases. Cancer 35:1430–1437, 1975.
11. Law DH, Liddle GW, Scott HW, Tauber SD: Ectopic Production of Multiple Hormones (ACTH, MSH and Gastrin) by a Single Malignant Tumor. N Engl J Med 273:292–296, 1965.

13. Low Grade Papillary Pancreatic Neoplasm in an Adolescent Female

MARILYN GREGORY PORTER, HENRY F. KROUS, ROBERT J. WEEDN and PERRY LAMBIRD

1. INTRODUCTION

We report an adolescent female with a rare papillary epithelial pancreatic neoplasm which is considered to have little malignant potential [1]. The tumor has not locally recurred or metastasized, but the patient experienced severe exocrine and endocrine pancreatic insufficiency following radical surgery including total pancreatectomy.

2. CASE REPORT

A 16-year old white female who had been in excellent health presented to her family physician complaining of an asymptomatic hard mass in the upper abdomen of three weeks duration. There was no family history of pancreatic neoplasia. Physical examination revealed a well-nourished, well-developed adolescent female with normal vital signs. A firm, large nontender mass was palpated in the right upper quadrant of the abdomen. The remainder of the physical examination was unremarkable. An upper gastrointestinal barium contrast study showed marked distortion of the duodenal C-loop by a tumor in the head of the pancreas. The tumor manifested marked vascularity by angiography. Serum carcinoembryonic antigen (CEA) was not detected pre- or post-operatively. At exploratory laporatomy, a large circumscribed 12 cm mass completely replacing the head of the pancreas was resected en bloc. The surgical procedure consisted of radical pancreaticoduodenectomy, splenectomy, cholecystectomy and partial gastrectomy. There were no immediate post-operative complications and she was discharged on the 15th post-operative day.

Over the next six months, she steadily lost weight and manifested brittle diabetes mellitus for which she was referred to Oklahoma Children's Me-

G. B. Humphrey et al. (eds.), Pancreatic Tumors in Children.
© 1982 Martinus Nijhoff Publishers, The Hague/Boston/London. ISBN-13:978-94-009-7617-7

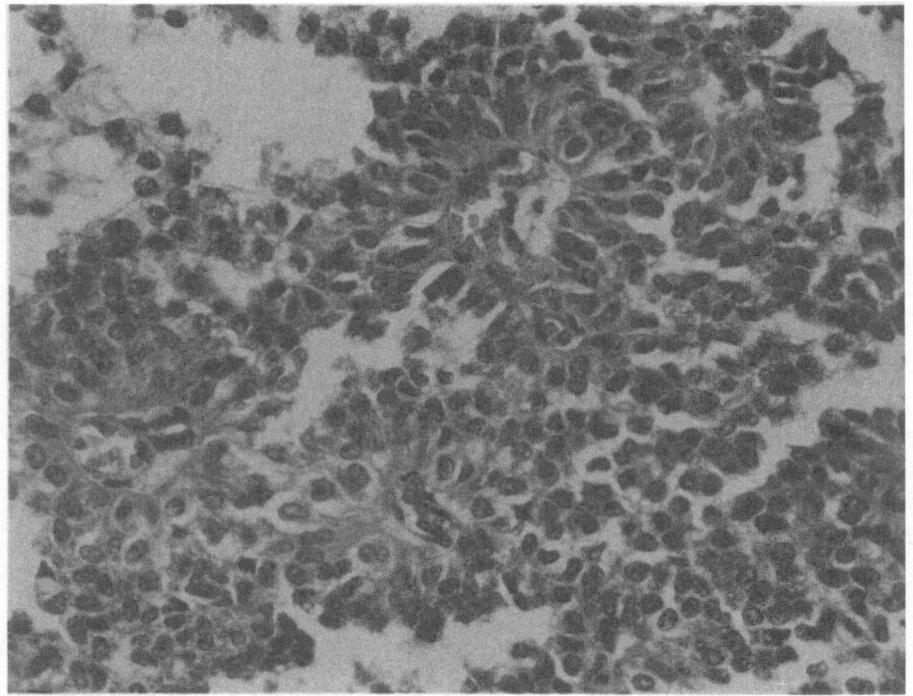

Figure 1. Papillary structures are created by tumor cells lining up and adherent to thin-walled blood vessels (H & E, × 100).

morial Hospital. Despite stabilization of diabetes, she continued to lose weight until she weighed 22.2 kg less than her pre-operative weight. The stool fat was 25 gm/24 hr (reference range less than 7 gm/24 hr), serum vitamin A 42 ng/dl (reference range 52–96 ng/dl), serum carotene 47 ng/dl (reference range 50–250 ng/dl), and serum 25-hydroxy vitamin D 10 ng/ml (reference range 10–55 ng/ml). Pancreatic enzyme replacement was increased as tolerated over the subsequent four months with a resultant weight gain of 5 kg and a reduction of fecal fat to 3.6 gm/24 hr. Additionally, cimetidine, medium chain triglycerides, safflower oil, and vitamin A, D, E and K supplements were administered.

The tumor has shown no evidence of recurrence or metastasis during the 27-month post-operative interval.

3. PATHOLOGY

An extensively necrotic circumscribed 12 cm tumor replaced the head of

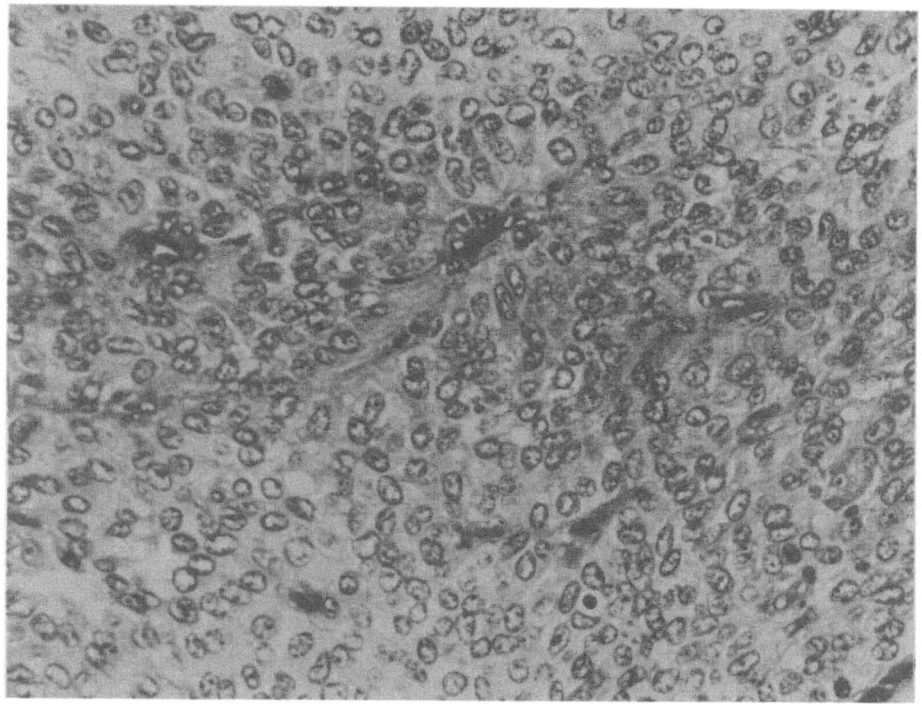

Figure 2. A compact cellular arrangement of tumor cells is interrupted by relatively numerous thin-walled blood vessels. Note that little pleomorphism is apparent (H & E, × 100).

the pancreas and extended into the peripancreatic soft tissue; however, the surgical margins were uninvolved. None of the regional lymph nodes contained tumor deposits.

Microscopically the partially encapsulated neoplasm had predominantly papillary architecture (Figure 1); however, other regions showed more compact cellular arrangement (Figure 2). The papillary structures were composed of columnar cells which were oriented along and around delicate blood vessels. The oval vesicular nuclei were generally placed peripheral to the base of the cell, and had prominent nuclear membranes with inconspicious nucleoli (Figure 3). The esosinophilic, finely granular cytoplasm of some cells tapered towards its attachment to or near thin-walled vessels. The cytologically benign tumor cells bore some resemblance to duct epithelium, however, convincing neoplastic ductal structures were not identified. Mitotic figures were extremely rare. Necrosis was most prominent in the central portion of the tumor. Histiocytes, some of which were multinucleate and contained cholesterol clefts, infiltrated the connective tissue at the

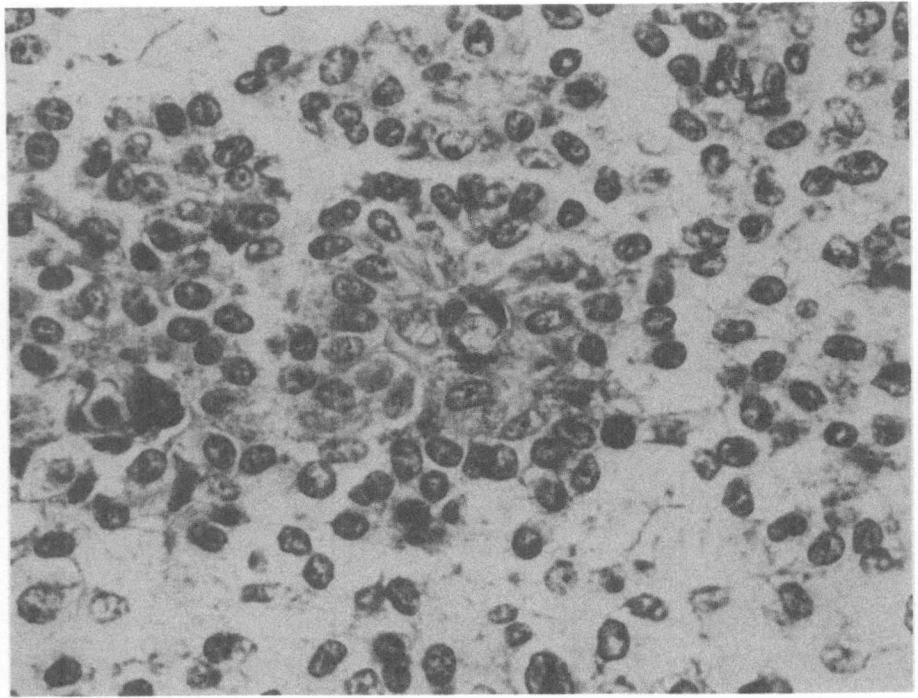

Figure 3. The oval vesicular nuclei are generally positioned in the apical portion of the tumor cells which showed tapering cytoplasmic attachments to a thin-walled vessel. Nucleoli are inconspicuous and minimal pleomorphism is present (H & E, × 250).

tumor periphery. Ductal structures and distorted islets were considered to represent compressed residual pancreas by the expanding tumor. Noncontiguous tumor deposits were not identified in regional soft tissue or extrapancreatic viscera.

Severe autolysis precluded detailed ultrastructural evaluation, however, zymogen and secretory granules were not identified.

The histologic diagnosis was papillary and solid pancreatic neoplasm.

4. DISCUSSION

Primary pancreatic tumors, whether benign or malignant, are rare in children [2]. During this period of life, the endocrine component is at greater risk of neoplastic transformation than the exocrine pancreas [3]; regarding the latter, ductal-derived tumors are more frequently encountered than those of acinar origin [4].

That the tumor of our patient is of probable ductal or ductular origin is based on circumstantial evidence. Pre-operative evidence of islet-cell hormonal imbalance was lacking and the tumor did not show light microscopic features characteristic of pancreatic endocrine tumors. Ultrastructural evaluation failed to disclose either islet-cell or zymogen granules, the latter of which should be identified in acinar derived tumors [4, 5, 6]. Other investigators have provided cogent arguments favoring ductal origin of such tumors based upon their ultrastructural similarity to pancreatic duct epithelium [1, 7, 8]. This hypothesis is perhaps further enhanced by the demonstration of neurosecretory granules in a papillary pancreatic tumor described by Schlosnagle and Campbell who summarize data that islets may have embryological origin from stem cells in duct epithelium [9].

Following surgical excision, neither radiation nor chemotherapy was administered. This decision was based on two factors. First, only one of nearly 60 patients reported with this tumor has experienced metastatic complications [1, 7, 8, 9]. On the other hand, patients have survived at least 21 years without recurrence [9]. Secondly, the tumor appeared histocytologically benign and was thought to be completely excised.

Demonstration of tumor recurrence can be difficult because of surgically distorted landmarks and absence of a proven biochemical marker such as CEA, galactosyl transferase isoenzyme II or pancreatic oncofetal antigen [11]. Despite its absence in our case, serum CEA was apparently not determined in those reported in the literature [1, 7, 8, 9, 10].

Compagno *et al.* abstracted 52 cases of this tumor from the files of the Armed Forces Institute of Pathology [1]. They found that these tumors preferentially affect women in their mid-twenties, are usually in the tail of the pancreas, and manifest very low grade malignancy, the latter determination of which was based upon a mean follow-up of 7.1 years.

The nutritional and metabolic derangements experienced by our patient illustrate the importance of medical management. Total pancreatectomy dictates continuous insulin and exocrine enzyme replacement while partial gastrectomy renders her vulnerable to the 'dumping syndrome' and malabsorption of iron, vitamin B12 and calcium.

REFERENCES

1. Compagno J, Oertel JE, Kremzar M: Solid and papillary epithelial neoplasm of the pancreas, probably of small duct origin: A clinical pathologic study of 52 cases. Lab Invest 40:248–249, 1979 (abstract).
2. Moynan RW, Neerhout RC, Johnson TS: Pancreatic carcinoma in childhood. J Pediatr 65:711–720, 1964.
3. Dehner LP: Pediatric surgical pathology, CV Mosby Co, 1975, pp 421–428.

186

4. Osborne BM, Culbert SJ, Cangir A, Mackay B: Acinar cell carcinoma of the pancreas in a 9-year old child: Case report with electron microscopic observations. South Med J 70:-370-372, 1977.
5. Taxy JB: Adenocarcinoma of the pancreas in childhood. Cancer 37:1508–1518, 1976.
6. Benjamin E. Wright DH: Adenocarcinoma of the pancreas of childhood: A report of 2 cases. Histopathology 4:87–104, 1980.
7. Hamoudi AB, Misugi K, Grosfeld JL, Reiner CB: Papillary epithelial neoplasm of pancreas in a child. Cancer 26:1126–1134, 1970.
8. Frantz VK: Tumors of the pancreas. In: Atlas of tumor pathology, VII, Fascicles 27 and 28. Washington, DC: Armed Forces Institute of Pathology, 1959, pp 32–33.
9. Boor PJ, Swanson MR: Papillary-cystic neoplasm of the pancreas. Am J Surg Pathol 3:-69–75, 1979.
10. Schlosnagle DC, Campbell WG Jr: The papillary and solid neoplasm of the pancreas: A report of 2 cases with electron microscopy, one containing neurosecretory granules. Cancer 47:2603–2610, 1981.
11. Ona FV, Zamcheck N, Dhar P, Moore T, Kupchik HZ: Carcinoembryonic antigen (CEA) in the diagnosis of pancreatic cancer. Cancer 31:324–327, 1973.

14. Cancer of the Pancreas in Children: Experience at the M.D. Anderson Hospital and Tumor Institute

NORMAN JAFFE and AYTEN CANGIR

Malignant neoplasms of the pancreas are uncommon in childhood. The purpose of this communication is to report the experience of the M.D. Anderson Hospital and Tumor Institute.

1. CARCINOMA OF THE PANCREAS

Only one child with carcinoma of the pancreas has been seen. This patient was the subject of the report published in March, 1977 [1]. He was a nine-year old boy who presented with abdominal pain and jaundice and was referred with a provisional diagnosis of lymphoma. Abdominal exploration revealed a normal pancreas and an exophytic mass within the leaves of the small bowel mesentery. The pancreas was described as normal to palpation.

Pathological examination revealed sheets of compactly arranged polyhedral cells with round central nuclei and rather scanty cytoplasm. There was no evidence of acinar formation. The impression was that the neoplasm was probably a small cell carcinoma, the origin of which could not be ascertained. Electron microscopy studies helped establish the diagnosis. The most significant feature was the presence of large secretory granules within the cytoplasm. The majority of the granules were over 1μ in diameter, each with a closely limiting unit membrane.

The patient responded initially to combination chemotherapy comprising actinomycin-D, 5-fluorouracil and cyclophosphamide. This was followed by radiation. However, this failed to maintain the response and an increase in the size of the tumor was noted. Radiation was discontinued and combination chemotherapy re-instated with only partial effect. A palpable abdominal mass was noted and needle aspiration of the peritoneal cavity revealed neoplastic cells. Other combinations of chemotherapy were introduced

G. B. Humphrey et al. (eds.), Pancreatic Tumors in Children.
© 1982 Martinus Nijhoff Publishers, The Hague/Boston/London. ISBN-13:978-94-009-7617-7

without response and the patient died two years after diagnosis. Autopsy revealed tumor localized to the abdominal cavity.

Electron microscopy was extremely helpful in clarifying the diagnosis. The large cytoplasmic aggregates of secretory material were typical of pancreatic acinar cells. Similar granules may be observed in serious cells of the salivary gland and in other salivary gland tumors. However, the granules in islet-cell neoplasms and other tumors are APUD (armine precursor uptake and decarboxylation) which are smaller.

A retrospective examination by light microscopy revealed occasional cells in the hematoxylin and eosin-stained sections in which acidophylic cytoplasmic granules similar to those seen in pancreatic acinar cells were present. These cells also suggested the diagnosis of acinar cell carcinoma. In this situation, a dimethylaminobenzaldhyde nitrite stain for tryptophan would be indicated.

ACKNOWLEDGEMENT

This work was supported in part by Grant No. CA 03713 from the National Institutes of Health.

REFERENCE

1. Osborne BM, Culbert SJ, Cangir A, Mackay B: Acinar cell carcinoma of the pancreas in a 9-year old child: case report with electron microscopic observations. South Med J 70:-370–372, 1977.

15. A Case of Metastatic Insulinoma in an Adolescent Girl

SHIAO Y. WOO, LUCIUS F. SINKS and PHILIP S. SCHEIN

1. INTRODUCTION

Pancreatic insulinoma, which arises from the B cells of islands of Langerhans, is a rare tumor affecting both sexes equally. Although the mean age at diagnosis is 42 years [1], the tumor has been reported in all age groups. In ten to fifteen percent of cases, the tumor is malignant and liver is the usual site of metastasis [2]. About ten percent of insulinomas occur as a component of multiple endocrine adenomatosis type I. The usual manifestation of insulinoma is neuroglycopenia. Extensive brain damage and neuropathy may result after frequent episodes of hypoglycemia. The diagnosis is established by demonstrating that the symptoms are caused by hypoglycemia and that there is excessive and inappropriate insulin secretion. The introduction of radioimmunoassay technique for determination of insulin and proinsulin levels has greatly facilitated the diagnosis of insulinoma.

This paper reports a case of metastatic malignant insulinoma in an adolescent girl seen in consultation at Georgetown University Hospital.

2. CASE HISTORY

B. O. was a 14½-year old white girl when she first presented with a five-week history of intermittent fever, abdominal pain, vomiting and episodes of grand mal seizures. She had been in good health prior to the illness. The abdominal pain occurred at the lower abdomen, was dull in character but with episodes of sharp pain and the pain had become more severe since the onset. She vomited only a few times with the abdominal pain. There was no history of diarrhea or constipation. She had at least one grand mal seizure preceded by cold sweat and tremors. She had also lost six pounds of weight in one month. There was no change in her appetite or menstrual patterns.

G. B. Humphrey et al. (eds.), Pancreatic Tumors in Children.
© 1982 Martinus Nijhoff Publishers, The Hague / Boston / London. ISBN-13:978-94-009-7617-7

Physical examination at that time revealed a thin girl without pallor or jaundice. Her heart rate was 100 per minute, regular. Blood pressure was 110/70 and respiratory rate 18 per minute. Her weight was 102 lbs and height 5'4". The only positive physical finding was an enlarged firm liver palpable 10 cm below right costal margin.

3. LABORATORY DATA

1) Hemoglobin 13.1 g/dl, hematocrit 39.7%, retic 0.67, WBC 8300/mm^3 (40% polys, 55% lymphs, 6% monos, 1% eos). Platelets 265,000/mm^3
2) Erythrocyte sedimentation rate 46 mm/hr
3) Bone marrow aspirate: normal marrow
4) Prothrombin time 11.9 sec (control 11.9 sec), partial thromboplastin time 37.6 sec (control 25–35 sec), fibrinogen 365 mg/dl
5) Uric acid 5.0 mg/dl   Albumin 4.4 g/dl
   Calcium 9.7 mg/dl   Bilirubin 0.1 mg/dl
   Phosphorus 4.3 mg/dl   SGOT 66 U/L
   Total protein 6.1 g/dl   SGPT 78 U/L
   LDH 167 U/L
   BUN 10 mg/dl
   Glucose (random) 65 mg/dl
6) Serum amylase 89 units/dl
   Urine amylase 99 units/2 hours
7) Alpha-fetoprotein: nondetectable
   Monospot: negative
   Australian antigen: negative
   ANA: negative
8) 5-Hydroxyindole acetic acid: 2.5 mg/dl (normal up to 10 mg/dl)
9) Gastrin level: 105 pg/ml (normal up to 300 pg/ml)
10) *Insulin levels:*

	Insulin mU/ml	Blood Sugar (mg/dl)
Patient	178.8	70 (10% glucose drip)
	66.0	45 (no glucose drip)
Mother (fasting)	11.5	98
Father (fasting)	26.4	90
Brother (fasting)	14.1	89
Sister (fasting)	10.2	80

11) *Column Fractionation on patient's sample:*
   insulin   =   19.2 uU/ml

proinsulin:

insulin std   =   50.7 uU/ml

proinsulin std = 269.3 uU/ml

% proinsulin   =   72.5

Comment: the insulin levels from the patient's sample are all markedly abnormal and consistent with the diagnosis of an insulinoma

12) CSF: WBC = 0, RBC = 0, sugar 43 mg/dl, protein 27 mg/dl. No malignant cells

13) EKG: normal

14) Chest X-ray: normal

15) Skeletal survey: normal

16) Upper GI Series: thickened folds of duodenal bulb especially in superior aspect; changes are consistent with localized pressure, wrapping around the duodenum or possibly a small para-aortic nodule. There is also external pressure on outer aspect of duodenal loop, probably from enlarged liver

17) Aortogram: marked encasement of proximal third of splenic artery is clearly demonstrated; findings characteristic of pancreatic neoplasm

18) Abdominal sonogram: hepatomegaly with irregular echoes, consistent with diffuse liver disease or metastasis. A very questionable area of mass in the region of the head of the pancreas is noted

19) Liver and spleen scan: the liver is enlarged with multiple space filling defects. The spleen appears normal in size. Impression: hepatomegaly with multiple metastases

20) Liver biopsy (needle): the hepatic lobular architecture as well as the hepatocytes are normal in appearance. Isolated islands to clumps of cells are scattered in the normal hepatic tissue. The cells in these islands are very uniform in size and shape and they have abundant eosinophilic cytoplasm and round nuclei. All these islands of cells are enclosed in a capsular space and they are reminiscent of islets of Langerhans in the pancreas. Special stain for beta granules is negative. Diagnosis: liver biopsies with metastatic tumor, comparable to insulinoma

4. TREATMENT

The patient was started on diazoxide 500 mg daily and phenobarbitol for seizure control. She was then seen in consultation at Georgetown University Medical Center and was placed on streptozotocin 1.5 g/m^2 and 5-FU 600 mg/m^2 weekly. Her treatment and follow-up were subsequently carried out by her physician in New York.

5. DISCUSSION

The occurrence of a typical hypoglycemic attack accompanied by a low blood glucose, and relief of symptoms by oral or intravenous glucose, constitutes the diagnostic 'Whipple's triad'. However, hypoglycemia may be absent at the time of examination of the patient, as was the case with this adolescent girl. Nevertheless, it was still possible to demonstrate an inappropriate elevation of the serum insulin and proinsulin levels. Occasionally, the secretion of insulin may be episodic and prolonged fasting (up to 72 hours) may be required to bring about hypoglycemia accompanied by inappropriately high plasma insulin levels. Other provocative tests, such as with the use of alcohol infusion, tolbutamide, glucagon, glucose, arginine, or cerulein may occasionally be of help but are now seldom used.

Localization of the primary tumor in the pancreas can be a difficult task especially when the tumor is small and nonmalignant. The tumor can also be multicentric. Selective arteriography and transhepatic pancreatic venous insulin sampling can be of great value though are by no means infallible. Computerized tomography and ultrasound may prove to be useful. Selenium scintiscan and ordinary tomogram are usually not helpful. In patients with obvious metastatic disease such as the case in this report, a liver biopsy will usually provide histologic confirmation of the diagnosis.

Surgical resection is the definitive treatment for both benign and malignant insulinomas. However, there are considerable differences of opinion as to what the appropriate procedure should be in many patients. The surgical decision is influenced by the size of the tumor in the pancreas, number of tumors and whether the tumor is localized pre-operatively or during surgery. Procedures such as enucleation, pancreatoduodenectomy, and progressive resection have all been used. In metastatic disease, radical surgery is usually not contemplated and the main objective of treatment is in the control of symptoms. Diazoxide, which inhibits secretion of insulin by the tumor, is useful in this regard.

Chemotherapy has been attempted. Objective response has been observed with streptozotocin [3], 5-fluorouracil [4], and tubercidin [4]. A recent study [5] showed that the combination of streptozotocin and 5-fluorouracil was superior to streptozotocin alone in overall rates of response (63 versus 36 percent), and possibly in duration of survival as well (median survival of 26 months versus 16½ months). The course of malignant insulinoma is characteristically indolent and survival from diagnosis of unresectable malignant disease to death frequently exceeds five years.

REFERENCES

1. Laurent J, Debry G, Floquest J: Surgical treatment of hypoglycemic tumors. Excerpta Medica: 78–83, 1971.
2. Scholz DA, Remine WH, Priestley JT: Hyperinsulinism: review of 95 cases of functioning pancreatic islet-cell tumors. Proc Staff Meet Mayo Clinic 35:545, 1960.
3. Broder LE, Carter SK: Islet-cell carcinoma (ICC): chemical features and results of therapy with streptozotocin (STR). Proc Amer Assoc Cancer Res 13:96, 1972.
4. Awrich A, Fletcher WS, Klotz JH, Minton JP, Hill GJ, Aust JB, Grage TD, Multhauf PM: 5-FU *versus* combination therapy with tubercidin, streptozotocin and 5-FU in the treatment of pancreatic carcinomas: COG protocol 7230. J Surg Oncol 12:267–273, 1979.
5. Moertel CG, Hanley JA, Johnson LA: Streptozotocin alone compared with streptozotocin plus fluorouracil in the treatment of advanced islet-cell carcinoma. N Engl J Med 303:1189–1194, 1980.

16. Experience with Endocrine and Exocrine Neoplasias in Children

ELAINE R. MORGAN, EDWARD S. BAUM and PATRICE M. WEST

Although carcinomas and adenocarcinomas are the most common histological types of cancer diagnosed in adults, they are extremely rare in children. These types of tumors comprise less than 5% of all malignancies diagnosed in children under the age of 15 years [1, 2]. Furthermore, cancer of glandular tissue (endocrine or exocrine) in children is exceedingly unusual [1]. However, tumors of glandular tissue, in a patient of any age, may be clinically significant, because of their metastatic potential, frequent association with hormone production, and resultant syndromes and complications.

Neoplasia, benign and malignant, involving the pancreas may be either hormone-functioning or nonfunctioning. These types of tumors are fairly common in adults, but extremely rare in children, with peak childhood incidence occurring in the preschool and early adolescent groups [3]. Functioning neoplasms may be either beta-type islet-cell tumors which may cause hypoglycemia or nonbeta-cell islet-cell tumors which are associated with the Zollinger-Ellison syndrome. The majority of these tumors are benign, however, occasionally malignant tumors of the pancreas may be of the functional variety. The remainder of the pancreatic carcinomas in children are nonfunctioning and are clinically most significant because of their malignancy potential. Fortunately, all pancreatic malignancies are very rare in children with only 25 cases having been reported up until 1970 [4].

Malignancy of other endocrine tissues is also quite unusual in children. Often, it may be difficult to determine whether a tumor is malignant or benign, since the histologic differentiation is not always clear [5]. Nonetheless, endocrine tumors present clinical problems whether benign or malignant because of their hormone production and consequent clinical syndromes.

There is very little information in the literature concerning the appropriate treatment of children with cancer of the endocrine glands. In general,

G. B. Humphrey et al. (eds.), Pancreatic Tumors in Children.
© 1982 Martinus Nijhoff Publishers, The Hague/Boston/London. ISBN-13:978-94-009-7617-7

Table 1. Clinical experience with endocrine and exocrine neoplasias

Patient	Date diagnosis	Sex	Age at diagnosis	Diagnosis	Presenting symptoms	Family picture	Rx	Comments
RV	1971	M	7 years	Pancreatic islet-cell adenoma	Tumor found at abdominal exploration $\bar{p}$ trauma	$\bar{O}$	One pre-operative course AMD subtotal pancreatectomy, one $\bar{p}$ op course AMD	Initial pathology islet-cell adenocarcinoma, subsequent review—adenoma, no evidence of disease
GE	1979	F	12 years	Pancreatic islet-cell carcinoma $\bar{c}$ hepatic metastases	Abdominal mass	$\bar{O}$	Biopsy; streptozotocin + 5-FU; Whipple procedure	Refused chemotherapy, $\bar{p}$ surgery. Expired 1 year $\bar{p}$ diagnosis

the approach has been surgical with a high cure rate in patients with endocrine malignancies who do not have metastases at diagnosis [3, 5]. Although pancreatic tumors have been approached surgically [4], the more aggressive pancreatic lesions, in children as in adults, are frequently not amenable to total surgical resection. Treatment of such tumors with chemotherapy has been attempted, most commonly using drugs such as 5-fluorouracil and streptozotocin with limited success. Radiotherapy does not appear to play a role in the treatment of pancreatic malignancy.

We have reviewed the tumor board records concerning all children who have presented with one of the above mentioned malignancies in the past years at Children's Memorial Hospital and the University of Chicago. The information concerning age at diagnosis, type of malignancy, family history, therapy and outcome are summarized in Table 1.

One of the patients received two courses of chemotherapy for what was initially believed to be a malignant lesion (RV). Review of the tissue revealed a benign appearing pancreatic islet-cell adenoma. The role of chemotherapy in this patient is unclear. The other patient, a young girl with nonfunctioning pancreatic carcinoma, presented with metastatic disease and subsequently died despite surgery and chemotherapy (GE).

Further review of other institutions' experience with these and other rare tumors. in children may yield insight into the appropriate diagnostic and therapeutic approach to such neoplasias.

REFERENCES

1. Sutow WW: General Aspects of Childhood Cancer. In: Clinical Pediatric Oncology, (2nd ed). Mosby CV, 1977, pp 1–15.
2. Silverberg E: Cancer Statistics. CA-A Cancer Journal for Clinicians 31:13–28, 1981.
3. Lane DM, Lonsdale D, Sutow WW: Tumors of the Gastrointestinal Tract. In: Clinical Pediatric Oncology, (2nd ed). Mosby CV, 1977, pp 553–561.
4. Grosfield JL, Clatworthy HW, Hamoudi AB: Pancreatic Malignancy in Childhood. Arch Surg 101:370–375, 1970.
5. Clayton GW: Tumors of the Endocrine Glands. In: Clinical Pediatric Oncology, (2nd ed). Mosby CV, 1977, pp 525–540.

17. Childhood Rare Endocrine Tumors

BARBARA CUSHING and A. JOSEPH BROUGH

Tumors of the endocrine system in the pediatric age group are a very small percentage of the total number of malignancies. Of these, germ cell tumors, some with endocrine function, and papillary or follicular thyroid carcinomas, associated with prior radiation exposure, are the most common. Tumors of the pancreas are exceedingly rare. The following chapter discusses the two cases presenting to Children's Hospital of Michigan from 1963 to 1981.

Carcinoma of the pancreas in a child has not been encountered in our institution. Both pancreatic tumors were benign islet-cell adenomas with hyperinsulinism. Both patients had a long history of recurrent episodes of hypoglycemia before the diagnosis was established; both continued with problems after partial pancreatectomies.

PANCREATIC ADENOMATOSIS

Case #1. Twelve-year old boy admitted for further evaluation of recently diagnosed hypoglycemia. The patient had an eighteen-month history of recurring episodes of weakness, dizziness, sweating, confusion, and loss of consciousness. Hypoglycemia secondary to insulin-secreting pancreatic tumor was suspected on the basis of the tolbutamide tolerance test. He was

Table 1. Two cases of pancreatic adenoma (benign) at Children's Hospital of Michigan (1963–1980)

Age	Sex	Race	Hormone activity	Therapy	Status
12 yr	M	Caucasian	Yes	Surgery	—
11 yr	M	Caucasian	Yes	Surgery	—

G. B. Humphrey et al. (eds.), Pancreatic Tumors in Children.
© *1982 Martinus Nijhoff Publishers, The Hague/Boston/London.* ISBN-13:978-94-009-7617-7

treated with diazoxide and although he became asymptomatic, random blood sugars were frequently low. Three years later, an exploratory laparotomy for partial pancreatectomy was done with removal of 80% of the body and tail of the pancreas. One macroscopic and numerous microscopic islet-cell adenomas were present. This has behaved clinically as a benign adenoma, however, hypoglycemia has persisted.

Case #2. Eleven-year old boy who presented with a three-year history of recurrent weakness, dizziness, mental confusion and generalized clonic seizures in the early morning. Anticonvulsants did not prevent episodic seizures. Twelve months prior to referral to CHM a diagnosis of hypoglycemia was made and triamcinolone was given with no improvement. On work-up at CHM, celiac axis angiography demonstrated mass in the tail of the pancreas. Leucine and tolbutamide tolerance tests were compatible with insulinoma. At laparotomy a 50% pancreatectomy and splenectomy were done. In the tail of the pancreas an encapsulated 4×3.5 cm nodule was found which represented islet-cell adenoma. Post-operatively the patient developed diabetes mellitus requiring insulin. He has had subsequent episodes of ketoacidosis and the impression is that the functioning adenoma masked the diabetes.

Two pre-adolescent males with very similar presentations have been managed at CHM. Both had prolonged, missed hypoglycemia and functioning insulinomas, with histologically benign islet-cell adenomas. One patient continued to be hypoglycemic following an 80% pancreatectomy for multiple adenomatosis and the other developed diabetes mellitus after a 50% pancreatectomy for a large solitary adenoma.

18. Overview of Childhood Pancreatic Tumors

THEODORE PYSHER, G. BENNETT HUMPHREY, STUART D. WILSON,

PHILIP S. SCHEIN, SARAH S. DONALDSON, RONALD M. BUKOWSKI

and JOHN KISSANE

1. INTRODUCTION

This volume includes several significant contributions to our understanding of pancreatic tumors in childhood. Tsukimoto has reviewed the Japanese literature [1] and Kissane the English literature, and Kissane presents a new pathological classification [2]. Horie has reiterated his view that infantile carcinoma of the pancreas arises from derivatives of the ventral pancreas [3], and Oertel and co-workers have provided a glimpse of their large collection of an unique group of pancreatic tumors that occur most often in young women [4]. There are also eight new cases reported from six institutions [5–11].

Pancreatic tumors are so rare in children that the information in current textbooks is of limited value [12–16]. Jones and Campbell's text is a notable exception and contains an excellent discussion of hyperinsulinemia and hypergastrinemia [17]. The remaining medical literature consists of case reports. The Third National Cancer Survey and the Cancer Surveillance Epidemiology and End Results Program (SEER) reported a zero average annual incidence rate from birth to 14 years. For white males 15 to 19 years of age the average annual incidence was less than 0.05 per 100,000 per year; for black females, 0.3 per year; and no cases were reported in white female or black male adolescents [18].

2. PRE-OPERATIVE EVALUATION

The pre-operative evaluation of nonfunctioning tumors is discussed by Falterman and Cohn [19] in their chapter, 'Pre-operative Evaluation of Pancreatic Tumors'. The approach to the child with a functioning tumor, such as Zollinger-Ellison syndrome (ZES), Cushing's syndrome and hypoglycemia

G. B. Humphrey et al. (eds.), Pancreatic Tumors in Children.
© 1982 Martinus Nijhoff Publishers, The Hague/Boston/London. ISBN-13:978-94-009-7617-7

are discussed and illustrated through case reports by Woo and co-workers and by Schmidt and Pysher [5, 8].

The value of the carcinoembryonic antigen (CEA) in pancreatic malignancies is discussed by Falterman and Cohn, and they do refer to Hunter's work with the pancreatic oncofetal antigen (POA) [20]. While CEA is commercially available, POA is not. However, Dr. Hunter is willing to evaluate serum from patients with pancreatic tumors for POA [20]. Five ml of frozen sera can be shipped to:

> Dr. Robert Hunter
> Clinical Immunology Laboratory
> Emory University Hospital
> 1364 Clifton Road
> Atlanta, GA 30322, U.S.A.

A letter describing the clinical and pathological presentation must accompany the sample.

A series of monoclonal antibodies raised against pancreatic antigens is also available. Individuals wishing to have pancreatic tumors evaluated with these reagents should contact Dr. R.S. Metzger at Duke University by telephone (919-684-3391) prior to the surgical excision of the tumor.

Since the submission of the Falterman and Cohn review, galactosyltransferase isoenzyme II has been reported to be a valuable marker in distinguishing benign from malignant pancreatic disease. However, this enzyme does not discriminate pancreatic from other gastrointestinal tumors [21]. It must be remembered that pancreatic tumors may produce more than one hormone and that they may be associated with the Type I multiple endocrine neoplasia syndrome [8, 22].

3. SURGERY

Smith has reviewed the surgical approach to a child with a nonfunctioning pancreatic tumor [23]. Of the functioning tumors, the Zollinger-Ellison syndrome (ZES) presents a particular challenge to the surgeon. The experience gained from the International ZES registry in Milwaukee, Wisconsin [24] is a valuable resource for clinicians faced with this condition. Cimetidine should be given pre-operatively to any patient with a known or suspected gastrin-secreting tumor. Total gastrectomy is the procedure of choice and partial gastrectomy is contraindicated [24].

4. PATHOLOGY OF EXOCRINE NEOPLASIAS

Kissane has suggested a new pathological classification for the 31 cases of pancreatic tumors of childhood reported in the literature [2]. In both Kissane's analysis and that of Tsukimoto, adenocarcinoma was the most prevalent among these rare malignant tumors.

The terminology of Kissane's review must be compared to the papers by Horie and by Tsukimoto as well as the series being collected by Oertel and co-workers [4]. Kissane prefers terminology that emphasizes the cell of origin. Thus, he divides the infantile carcinoma of the pancreas into two categories: the pleomorphic type of presumed acinar origin and the solid and papillary type of presumed ductal origin. Others have proposed that all carcinomas of the pancreas in childhood originate from duct epithelium [25]. Horie terms these lesions pancreatoblastoma and equates them with nephroblastoma, hepatoblastoma and pneumoblastoma. He also places prognostic significance on whether the tumor originates from the dorsal or ventral anlage [3]. Horie's pancreatoblastoma (of both dorsal and ventral anlage) are contained within Kissane's pleomorphic type, and both authors review some of the same case material. There is also some overlap in the material quoted by Tsukimoto. The series of adolescents and adults currently being evaluated by Oertel and co-workers are histologically similar to the case reported by Hamoudi et al. in 1970 and would be classified as solid and papillary type by Kissane.

5. PATHOLOGY OF ENDOCRINE NEOPLASIAS

Kissane's classification does not include endocrine tumors of the pancreas, but some discussion of the pathology of endocrine tumors is included in the report of Schmidt and Pysher [8].

Routine histologic study of islet-cell tumors correlates poorly with the functional status of a tumor or its subsequent biologic behavior [26]. Electron microscopy can add precision to the diagnosis—the presence of secretory granules establishing an endocrine origin [27], but only a few hormones are stored in ultrastructurally unique granules [28]. Correlation of products with morphology is best achieved by histochemical or, preferably, immunocytochemical means. Tissue culture, as described by Kissane, is an exciting avenue for future investigation, but the ability of this technique to reliably differentiate islet-cell tumors from those of parenchymal origin remains to be proven [2].

Much of the nosologic difficulty with pancreatic tumors in childhood derives from the disputed embryology of islet cells. A common origin for peptide-hormone secreting cells had been suspected for many years because of striking morphologic similarities, under both normal and neoplastic conditions, among these widely distributed cells. Furthermore, such neoplasms produced a variety of endocrine symptoms, often not at all related to the gland of origin. In 1969, A.G.E. Pearse demonstrated that many peptide-secreting endocrine cells, including islet cells, shared a number of cytochemical reactions and ultrastructural features [29]. He proposed a neural crest origin for all of these cells and created the terms APUD (from the ability of the cells for Amine Precursor Uptake and Decarboxylation) for the cells themselves, APUDOMA for tumors derived from any member of the group, and neurocristopathy for disorders of the group in general.

Though belonging to Pearse's APUD system by virtue of their cytochemistry, the neural crest origin of islet cells is disputed. Removal of the neural fold from nine-day old rat embryoes does not preclude development of secretory granules in pancreatic islets [30]. An earlier migration cannot be excluded, and in fact, is invoked by neurocristopathists [31], but others deny that it ever occurs [32]. The progenitors of islet cells are thus at least closely intermingled with, if not identical with ductular cells from early gestation. Therefore, a tumor of primitive ductal epithelium might well have features of exocrine or endocrine cells, or even both. Study of undifferentiated tumors suggests that this identity extends to the ultrastructural level [33]. Until this issue is settled, tissue culture studies must be interpreted with caution. *In vitro* differentiation could proceed in either direction, depending upon culture conditions.

Nieuwenhuijzen Kruseman, *et al.* [34] correlated histology and immunocytochemistry. They found that glucagon-producing tumors formed thin ribbons of cells, while tumors composed of insulin- or gastrin-producing cells usually formed solid nests. However, clinical and morphological correlation has not been so precise in other studies. Cubilla and Hajdu reviewed 30 cases of malignant islet-cell tumors accumulated over 25 years at the Memorial Sloan-Kettering Cancer Center [26]. Patients ranged from 8 to 76 years of age, with an average of 44 years, and the only child was an 8-year old girl. Twelve of the 30 patients evidenced endocrine abnormalities, including hypoglycemia, hyperglycemia and the Zollinger-Ellison syndrome, but there were no consistent gross or histologic differences between functioning and nonfunctioning tumors. Furthermore, size of tumor, local infiltration, and vascular invasion did not correlate with the presence of metastases at the time of diagnosis or during the subsequent course. These authors concluded that their study confirmed '... that the ultimate criterion that defines the nature of islet-cell tumors is the documentation of metastases.'

The status of clinical-morphological correlation has been recently reviewed by Bordi and Tardini [28], Larsson [30], and by Klöppel and co-workers [35]. Ultrastructural identification of secretory granules allows classification as an endocrine tumor, and in some cases, the granules sufficiently

Table 1. Commercially available hormones of relevance to evaluation of children with pancreatic tumors

Insulin
Glucagon
Somatomedin
ACTH
Gastrin
VIP

resemble those found in normal A, B, D, PP, EC or G cells that functional correlation is possible. Problems arise, however, when granules are small (100–200 nm) because several clinical syndromes have been associated with such granules; when cells are poorly granulated; or when more than one type of granule is identified within a cell or in different cells from various regions of the tumor. Immunocytochemistry offers the advantages of a larger (and presumably more representative) sample, as well as identification of the product. This would be desirable in all cases, but is essential when islet-cell tumors are associated with products not normally produced in the pancreas, as one must demonstrate that the proliferation of islet cells is indeed the source rather than the result of the ectopic hormone [28]. Moreover, biochemical studies can be done on frozen tumor and/or tumor cell cultures. Final classification should come from correlation of clinical symptoms and endocrinologic investigations with the results of the broadest possible spectrum of morphologic, immunologic and biochemical tests. Commercially available serum biochemical assays are listed in Table 1.

6. CLINICAL CLASSIFICATION AND PROGNOSIS

Four of the histopathologic types of pancreatic carcinoma appear to have clinical significance—adenocarcinoma, pleomorphic type and solid and papillary types of exocrine tumors, and islet-cell tumors. The acinar type of adenocarcinoma will not be discussed further as there is only a single case report.

In order to obtain as many cases as possible in each category, we will pool the data from the Japanese (Horie and Tsukimoto) and American (Kissane) reviews, and from the institutions submitting case reports for this volume. Acknowledging the risk of drawing conclusions based on patients from different series lacking a central pathological review, and of the differing environmental and/or genetic factor, we still think useful clinical knowledge may be gained from such an approach.

206

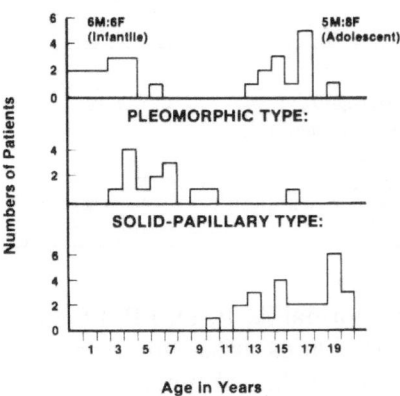

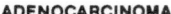

ADENOCARCINOMA

6M:6F (Infantile)   5M:8F (Adolescent)

PLEOMORPHIC TYPE:

SOLID-PAPILLARY TYPE:

Numbers of Patients

Age in Years

Figure 1. Adenocarcinoma.

6.1. Adenocarcinoma

This type appears to have a bimodal age distribution in the pediatric age group. The first is a childhood or infantile clustering of 12 cases, 11 of which occurred during the first five years of life and the 12th case at age six. No cases occurred between the 7th to the 12th year of life. The second group includes 13 adolescents (Figure 1). This bimodal age distribution has been reported by others [36]. The sex ratio in the childhood group is equal—six males and six females. It is interesting to speculate what role a perinatal exposure to an oncogenic agent might have played in the etiology of this infantile subgroup. The adolescent group probably represents the tail of the more typical adult pancreatic carcinoma. The sex distribution for the adolescent group was five males and eight females. In any case, adenocarcinoma, whether in an infant or adolescent, carries an extremely poor prognosis. All patients except three have died of their primary tumors. One of those three has been under observation for only eight months; in a second, the tumor was an incidental finding in an autopsy for leukemia; and the third is alive and well 18 years after surgery [11]. Even with complete surgical excision, some form of post-surgical therapy seems warranted in this group of patients.

6.2. Pleomorphic Type (Acinar Differentiation)

This is one of two subcategories in Kissane's classification of immature pancreatic malignancies. Horie discusses this same tumor as a pancreato-blastoma. If one eliminates the duplication of case material between Kissane and Horie, there are 14 such tumors reported in this volume. All but one of these, a 16-year old female, fall in the age range of three to ten years.

There were eight males and six females. The group has a poor prognosis: five of fourteen patients are already dead and the period of observation for several of the survivors is rather short. Kissane does not further subdivide this group, but Horie does and feels that his subdivision has prognostic significance.

6.3. Solid and Papillary Type (Ductal Differentiation)

Oertel and co-workers have collected 26 cases, 20 years old or younger, and Kissane includes four others in his review. Two of the four patients reported by Kissane are dead. None of the 26 adolescents described by Oertel and co-workers have died of metastasis, and they feel that this is a very low grade malignancy. Of the adult patients followed by Oertel and co-workers (not reported here), at least one has died from tumor and several are alive with metastases.

6.4. Functioning and Nonfunctioning Islet-Cell Tumors

The literature on these tumors is very difficult to evaluate if ultrastructure was not reported [27]. Further, many pathologists do not classify islet-cell tumors as malignant or benign on morphologic criteria. Four nonfunctioning islet-cell tumors are included in this volume—three reported by Tsukimoto and one by Morgan and co-workers [1, 9]. Two of the patients are dead, one is alive in relapse 2½ years after surgery and one is apparently tumor-free with only a 10-month follow-up. This suggests a poor prognosis.

A second group of the islet-cell tumors are those associated with clinical syndromes [37, 38]. Zollinger-Ellison syndrome (ZES), hypoglycemia and Cushing's syndrome have been described in children. While an occasional child will present with diarrhea (i.e., Horie's series), it appears that pancreatic neoplasias directly causing diarrhea are extremely rare in children. In one series of 28 children, none presented with diarrhea [39].

There are more cases of ZES available for analysis than other functional islet-cell tumors because of the International ZES registry at Milwaukee. In 1965, Wilson reported 15 cases in whom the first surgical procedure occurred on or before the 16th birthday [24]. In 13 of these cases, the tumor was classified as malignant and in 11, there were metastases to the liver, lymph nodes or duodenum (in decreasing order of frequency). Eight of the 13 patients had less than a total gastrectomy. Six of these eight had succumbed to complications of continued gastric hypersecretion. One of the two living patients underwent total gastrectomy and was alive at the last follow-up. The other patient had a subtotal gastrectomy and has been lost to follow-up [40]. Seven children underwent total gastrectomy and all were alive at the time of the 1965 report. Subsequently, one patient (#9) died approximately 15 years after total gastrectomy, presumably a tumor-related death [40]. There have been five additional children entered into the International ZES registry since 1965. Wilson's experience has underscored the high incidence of multiple tumors within the pancreas and the presence of metastatic disease at diagnosis. Elevated gastrin levels have been observed for periods of five to eleven years after surgery, presumably due to residual metastatic disease.

Thus, islet-cell tumors are compatible with a prolonged survival. However, children who present with ulcers in the duodenum, jejunum or antrum should be evaluated for ZES, have serum gastrin levels determined and, if elevated, be further evaluated for hepatic metastases and a pancreatic tumor. The one case reported in this volume by Schmidt and Pysher [8] resembled a mixed endocrine islet-cell tumor with Cushing's syndrome being the predominant clinical feature. This case, however, does emphasize the need to evaluate patients for more than one hormone. Only one patient in Wilson's report has a 'familial' gastrinoma, i.e., MEN I. It should be emphasized that we should not group these familial patients with the 'sporadic' form of gastrinoma. The 'sporadic' form has no family history of endocrine disorders and no other endocrine systems are involved. The patients with MEN I invariably have a positive family history. Further considerations of the treatment and natural history of gastrinomas in MEN is presented in Volume 3 of this series [41].

In children, malignant insulin-secreting tumors are much rarer than malignant gastrin-secreting tumors. Benign insulin-secreting tumors are not uncommon. Welch has collected 54 cases of benign insulinomas in children, 22 of whom were less than two years of age [30]. The remaining 32 cases were more or less randomly distributed within the childhood years [39]. Jones and Campbell describe a case in which an insulinoma may have transformed into a nonsecreting carcinoma [17]. These authors refer to three additional cases of malignant beta-cell tumors. The case report by Woo and co-workers in this volume provides an excellent description of the evaluation of patients with suspected insulinomas and includes guidelines for the management and chemotherapy [5].

Finally, it must be remembered that not all abdominal tumors presenting with Cushing's syndrome will be of adrenal origin. Schmidt and Pysher's case, albeit a rare event, must be kept in mind when evaluating a patient presumed to have a neoplasm of the adrenal cortex [8].

7. CHEMOTHERAPY

The post-operative management of tumors of the pancreas should depend upon the histology of the tumor. Recommendations are made for the four groups of tumors discussed above.

7.1. Adenocarcinoma

Even though adenocarcinoma can be divided into infantile and adolescent (adult) subgroups, the same therapeutic recommendations are made for both subgroups because both have a poor prognosis. Recently, there has been some small success in treating this malignancy with multiple drug chemotherapy. Whether as adjuvant therapy or treatment of residual or metastatic disease, there are three regimens from the adult literature that ought to be considered for children: SMF (streptozotocin, mitomycin C, 5-fluorouracil), FAM (5-fluorouracil, adriamycin, metomycin C) and FAM-S (FAM plus streptozotocin). The doses and schedules for these regimens vary as does the toxicity [42, 43]. The first two regimens have been under evaluation for a number of years so more is known about their toxicity and relative efficacy. In most series, both regimens have equivalent efficacy, however, one trial suggests that SMF is superior to FAM. FAM is better tolerated since renal toxicity, secondary to streptozotocin, is a potential complication of the SMF regimen. Since children generally tolerate streptozotocin better than adults, this may not be a problem. One of the co-authors recommends SMF as preferred therapy, adding that renal function should be monitored closely, and if toxicity develops, streptozotocin should be discontinued and adriamycin substituted (or use FAM). Another co-author would recommend FAM-S due to encouraging early results which included a 48% response rate with this four-drug combination [43]. Tsukimoto, in his report, comments that a few patients responded to cytoxan, vincristine and mitomycin C; but, unfortunately, does not identify which tumors responded to this three-drug combination [1].

7.2. Pleomorphic Type

Careful observation is clearly warranted; however, more experience will be necessary before adjuvant therapy can be recommended.

7.3. Solid and Papillary type

If Oertel's experience is correct, this tumor is a low grade malignancy, and observation is all that is indicated.

7.4. Islet-Cell Tumors

All such tumors are potentially malignant. A nonfunctioning tumor may have a particularly poor prognosis, but again, more cases must be evaluated before adjuvant chemotherapy can be recommended. In the functional tumors, surgical management has already been discussed. Chemotherapeutic recommendations are outlined in the report of Woo et al. [5].

8. RADIATION THERAPY

There is inadequate experience with the use of therapeutic radiation in the treatment of childhood pancreatic tumors from which to draw firm recommendations regarding its use in children. However, utilizing the pathological categorization proposed by Kissane, we can assume that the most common subtype of childhood pancreatic carcinoma, the adenocarcinoma, which is morphologically indistinguishable and has a similar biologic pattern as the adult form, may respond to radiation in a similar fashion.

Experience with radiation therapy for pancreatic adenocarcinomas in adults demonstrates that therapeutic radiation given with curative intent, is most effective among those patients who following surgical exploration and resection are known to have localized or regional disease. These cancers are not radioresistant as previously thought. They do, however, require high radiation doses for local control. This requires careful localization procedures and the use of beam shaping devices, as the pancreas is located in close proximity to other structures whose radiosensitivity limits the dose of radiation which can be delivered by external beam megavoltage irradiation.

Development of high-energy photon and electron beams may make it possible to deliver large tumor doses to the pancreas while sparing sensitive adjacent normal tissues. Furthermore, use of interstitial irradiation by the direct application of radioactive sources implanted into the primary tumor and surrounding bed allows delivery of high radiation doses to a precisely defined small volume. Further exploration of the use of radiation combined with radiation sensitizers may also significantly increase the effective radiation dose which may be delivered to a localized pancreatic tumor. Recent reviews of the experiences in adults demonstrate that high dose external beam radiotherapy does impact on local control and survival rates [44]. Research protocols incorporating the newer aspects of administration of radiotherapy with chemotherapy are being developed in therapeutic programs for adults [45]. It is possible that those protocols found to be effective for treatment of adenocarcinomas of adults can then be effectively utilized in the treatment of pancreatic adenocarcinomas of children.

For pancreatic carcinomas which are found to be widespread at the time of presentation, the role of radiotherapy is limited to one of palliation of symptomatic masses, relief of pain and obstructive jaundice.

The embryonal form of pancreatic childhood neoplasms, the pancreatico-blastoma, may be analogous to solid embryonic tumors of childhood in other sites. If so, it is possible that radiotherapy may be a possible effective modality for treatment of localized disease.

9. FOR FUTURE CASES

We encourage clinicians to register chemotherapeutic trials undertaken with adenocarcinoma of the pancreas with our editorial offices. Flow sheets and/or an informal letter summarizing results can be forwarded to our offices and will be shared with other clinicians upon request. Address correspondence to:

Editorial Offices, *Pediatric Oncology*
c/o G.B. Humphrey
Oklahoma Children's Memorial Hospital
940 N.E. 13th
Oklahoma City, OK 73104, U.S.A.
1-800-522-0211

REFERENCES

1. Tsukimoto I, Tsuchida M: Pancreatic carcinoma in children in Japan — Review of the Japanese literature. In: This volume.
2. Kissane JM: Tumors of the exocrine pancreas in childhood. In: This volume.
3. Horie A: Pancreatoblastoma. Histopathologic criteria based up on a review of six cases. In: This volume.
4. Oertel JE, Mendelsohn G, Compagno J: Solid and papillary epithelial neoplasms of the pancreas. In: This volume.
5. Woo SY, Sinks LF, Schein PS: A case of metastatic insulinoma in an adolescent girl. In: This volume.
6. Jaffe N, Cangir A: Cancer of the pancreas in children: Experience at the M.D. Anderson Hospital and Tumor Institute. In: This volume.
7. Raney RB, Meadows AT, D'Angio GJ: Personal communication.
8. Schmidt JH, Pysher TJ: Ectopic Cushing's syndrome in an adolescent. In: This volume.
9. Morgan ER, Baum ES, West PM: Experience with endocrine and exocrine neoplasias in children. In: This volume.
10. Cushing B, Brough AJ: Childhood rare endocrine tumors. In: This volume.
11. Porter MG, Krous H, Weedn RJ, Lambird P: Low grade papillary pancreatic neoplasm in an adolescent female. In: This volume.
12. Sutow WW: Malignant solid tumors in children. A review. New York: Raven Press, 1981.
13. Al-Rashid RA: Pediatric cancer chemotherapy. New York: Medical Examination Publishing Co, 1979.
14. Altman AJ, Schwartz AD: Malignant diseases of infancy, childhood and adolescence. Philadelphia, London, Toronto: W.B. Saunders Co, 1978.
15. Sutow WW, Vietti TJ, Fernbach DJ (eds): Clinical pediatric oncology. Saint Louis: CV Mosby Co, 1977.
16. Bloom HJG, Lemerle J, Neidhardt MK, Voûte PA (eds): Cancer in children. Clinical management. Berlin, Heidelberg, New York: Springer-Verlag, 1975.
17. Jones PG, Campbell PE (eds): Tumours of infancy and childhood. Oxford, London, Edinburgh, Melbourne: Blackwell Scientific Publications, 1976.

212

18. Berg JW, Connelly RR: Updating the epidemiologic data on pancreatic cancer. Semin Oncol 6:275–284, 1979.
19. Falterman KW, Cohn I: Pre-operative evaluation of pancreatic tumors. In: This volume.
20. Gelder FB, Reese CJ, Moossa AR, Hall T, Hunter R: Purification, partial characterization, and clinical evaluation of a pancreatic oncofetal antigen. Cancer Res 38:313–324, 1978.
21. Podolsky DK, McPhee MS, Alpert E, Warshaw AL, Isselbacher KJ: Galactosyltransferase isoenzyme II in the detection of pancreatic cancer: Comparison with radiologic, endoscopic, and serologic tests. N Engl J Med 304:1313–1318, 1981.
22. Majewski JT, Wilson SD: The MEN-I syndrome: An all or none phenomenon? Surgery 86:475–484, 1979.
23. Smith EI: Surgical therapy in pancreatic malignancies in children. In: This volume.
24. Wilson SD, Ellison EH: Total gastric resection in children with the Zollinger-Ellison syndrome. Arch Surg 91:165–173, 1965.
25. Taxy JB: Adenocarcinoma of the pancreas in childhood. Report of a case and review of the English language literature. Cancer 37:1508–1518, 1976.
26. Cubilla AL, Hajdu SI: Islet cell carcinoma of the pancreas. Arch Pathol 99:204–207, 1975.
27. Vozis EE, Pritzker KPH: Pancreatic islet cell tumor in childhood. Can Med Assoc J 122:435–438, 1980.
28. Bordi C, Tardini A: Electron microscopy of islet cell tumors. In: Progress in surgical pathology, Volume I, Fenoglio CM, Wolff M (eds). New York: Masson, 1980, pp 135–155.
29. Pearse AGE: The cytochemistry and ultrastructure of polypeptide hormone-producing cells (the APUD series) and the embryologic, physiologic and pathologic implications of the concept. J Histochem Cytochem 17:303–313, 1969.
30. Rutter JW, Pictet RL, Harding JD, et al.: An analysis of pancreatic development; role of mesenchymal factor and other extracellular factors. In: Molecular control of proliferation and differentiation, Papaconstantinou E (ed). New York: Academic Press, 1978, pp 205–227.
31. Larsson L-I: Endocrine pancreatic tumors. Hum Pathol 9:401–416, 1978.
32. Andrew A: Further evidence that enterochromaffin cells are not derived from the neural crest. J Embryol Exp Morphol 31:589–598, 1974.
33. Capella C, Solcia E, Frigerio B, et al.: The endocrine cells of the pancreas and related tumours. Ultrastructural study and classification. Virchows Arch A (Pathol Anat) 373:327–352, 1977.
34. Nieuwenhuijzen Kruseman AC, Knijnenburg G, Brutel de la Rivière G, Bosman FT: Morphology and immunohistochemically-defined endocrine function of pancreatic islet cell tumours. Histopathology 2:389–399, 1978.
35. Klöppel G, Seifert G, Heith PhV: Endokrine Pankreastumoren: Morphologie und Syndrome. Dtsch Med Wochenschr 44:1571–1577, 1979.
36. Benjamin E, Wright DH: Adenocarcinoma of the pancreas of childhood: A report of two cases. Histopathology 4:87–104, 1980.
37. Schein PS, DeLellis RA, Kahn CR, Gorden P, Kraft AR: Islet cell tumors: Current concepts and management. Ann Intern Med 79:239–257, 1973.
38. Katz R, Fischmann AB, Galotto J, Guccio JG, Higgins GA, Ortega LG, West WH, Recant L: Necrolytic migratory erythema, presenting as candidiasis, due to a pancreatic glucagonoma. Cancer 44:558–563, 1979.
39. Welch KJ: The pancreas. In: Pediatric surgery, Vol 2, Ravitch MM, Welch KJ, Benson CD, Aberdeen E, Randolph JG (eds). Chicago, London: Year Book Medical Publishers, Inc, 1979, pp 857–877.
40. Wilson SD: Personal communication.

41. Humphrey GB, Pysher T, Holcombe J, Rowsey JJ, Burris TE, Lemerle J, Wilson SD, Carney JA, Schimke RN: Overview of the multiple endocrine neoplasia syndromes in infancy and childhood. In: Pediatric Oncology, Vol 3 (in press).
42. Smith FP, Schein PS: Chemotherapy of pancreatic cancer. Semin Oncol 6:368–377, 1979.
43. Bukowski RM, Schacter LP, Groppe CW, Hewlett JS, Weick JK, Livingston RB: Phase II trial of 5-fluorouracil, adriamycin, mitomycin C and streptozotocin (FAM-S) in pancreatic carcinoma. Cancer (in press).
44. Borgelt BB, Dobelbower RR, Strubler KA: Betatron therapy for unresectable pancreatic cancer. A preliminary report. Am J Surg 135:76–80, 1978.
45. Dobelbower RR: The radiotherapy of pancreatic cancer. Semin Oncol 6:378–389, 1979.

SUBJECT INDEX

Acanthosis nigricans, 83
Acromegaly, 82, 83
ACTH (*see* Hormone, adrenocorticotropic)
Actinomycin D, 47, 187
ADCC: activity may be augmented by NK cells,
    16
    chemotherapy, 208-209
    predominates in childhood, 178, 205
    prognosis, 206
    response to radiation, 209-210
    treatment by resection, 147
Adenoma
    acinar, 104
    hyperparathyroidism, 85
    islet cell, 89, 197, 199-200
    microcystic, 104
Adenosine deaminase: activity reduced in
    human colon cancer cells by DMF, 50
Adenocystoma: papillary, 105
Adriamycin, 15, 209
Age, effects of: growth of transplantable
    tumors in nude mice, 5
Aldosteronoma, 86
ALL (*see* Leukemia, acute lymphoblastic)
Alpha fetoprotein: used for diagnosis of pan-
    creatic carcinoma, 132
Anemia: Fanconi's, 31, 37
Aneuploidy, 32-33
Angiography: role in diagnosis of pancreatic
    carcinoma, 137
ANLL (*see* Leukemia, acute nonlymphocytic)
Anti-asialo GM1: administered to nude mice, 7
Antigen
    carcinoembryonic, 132, 202
    pancreatic oncofetal, 132, 202
APL (*see* Leukemia, acute promyelocytic)
Armed Forces Institute of Pathology, 105, 159,
    185

Asialo GM1: expressed by NK cell-containing
    populations, 7
Aspirin
    inhibitor of prostaglandin synthesis, 9
    restores normal levels of NK activity in
        murine sarcoma virus treated mice, 17
Assay: microleukocyte adherence inhibition
    used for diagnosis of pancreatic carcinoma,
    132-133
Ataxia-telangiectasia, 31, 36-37
Auer rods, 61, 62

Biopsy: role in study of pancreatic lesions, 137-
    138, 145
Butyric acid: induces differentiation of leuke-
    mia cells, 47

Calcitonin
    secreted by pheochromocytomas, 88
    secreted by somatostatinomas, 90
Cancer
    colon: effects of maturational agents, 48-50
    lung: cilia formation caused by DMSO, 48
Cancer Surveillance Epidemiology and End
    Results Program, 201
Carcinoma
    acinar, 113, 114, 115, 119
    adenosquamous, 122
    adrenal-cortical, 87
    breast, 87
    lysed by NK cells, 10
    pancreas, 106-106, 187-188, 197
        age of patients, 106
        classification, 108
        diagnosis, 107
        four histopathologic types, 205
        immunology, 132-133
        incidence in Japan, 149